Drug Treatments and Dementia

Bradford Dementia Group Good Practice Guides

*Now under the editorship of Murna Downs, this series constitutes a set of accessible, jargon-free good practice guides for the carers of people with dementia. Reflecting the group's commitment to the person-centred approach to dementia, the series draws on both experience in practice and the latest research in the fields of dementia and dementia care. **Murna Downs** is Chair in Dementia Studies at Bradford University and the head of the Bradford Dementia Group. Before taking up her present position she directed the Centre for Social Research on Dementia at Stirling University.*

Primary Care and Dementia
Steve Iliffe and Vari Drennan
ISBN 1 85302 997 1

Training and Development for Dementia Care Workers
Anthea Innes
ISBN 1 85302 761 8

Social Work and Dementia
Good Practice and Care Management
Margaret Anne Tibbs
ISBN 1 85302 904 1

of related interest

Including the Person with Dementia in Designing and Delivering Care
'I Need to Be Me!'
Elizabeth Barnett
Foreword by Mary Marshall
ISBN 1 85302 740 5

Understanding Dementia
The Man with the Worried Eyes
Richard Cheston and Michael Bender
ISBN 1 85302 479 1

Hearing the Voice of People with Dementia
Opportunities and Obstacles
Malcolm Goldsmith
Preface by Mary Marshall
ISBN 1 85302 406 6

Bradford Dementia Group Good Practice Guides

Drug Treatments and Dementia

Stephen Hopker

Jessica Kingsley Publishers
London and Philadelphia

The right of Stephen Hopker to be identified as author of this work has been asserted by him in accordance with the Copyright, Designs and Patents Act 1988.

First published in the United Kingdom in 1999 by
Jessica Kingsley Publishers Ltd,
116 Pentonville Road, London
N1 9JB, England
and
325 Chestnut Street,
Philadelphia PA 19106, USA.

www.jkp.com

Second impression 2001

Library of Congress Cataloging in Publication Data
A CIP catalog record for this book is available from the Library of Congress

British Library Cataloguing in Publication Data
Hopker, Stephen
Drug treatments and dementia. – (Bradford Dementia Group ; 1)
1. Dementia – Chemotherapy
I. Title
616.8'3

ISBN 1 85302 760 X

Printed and Bound in Great Britain by
Athenaeum Press, Gateshead, Tyne and Wear

Contents

Preface

I write this preface with mixed feelings. On the one hand, I am naturally pleased to introduce this book, which I hope will be of value in helping people from many backgrounds to understand more about drug treatments for persons with dementia, including the several areas of debate, and even controversy, which surround this topic.

Yet – I should not be writing this preface at all. Its author should have been Professor Tom Kitwood, holder of the Alois Alzheimer Chair at the University of Bradford. Tragically he died in November 1998, very unexpectedly, within days of a prize-giving ceremony for what may come to be seen as a particularly important work, *Dementia Reconsidered: The Person Comes First* (Kitwood 1997). It was through Tom's kind invitation that I came to write this book, which is an early member of a series focusing on dementia care: Tom was to be the series editor.

I have been very fortunate in that Tom had already performed the main editorial task in respect of this book, providing not only notes on grammar and style, but also guidance in direction: in particular, to develop a strand of thinking already present in my first draft, namely the vital necessity of keeping a focus on the person affected by dementia, rather than just the disease: that is, to retain a humanitarian framework which goes beyond purely medical or scientific ways of thinking.

I understand that, in seeking a successor to Professor Kitwood as leader of the Bradford Dementia Group, one of the responsibilities of the post will be to continue the editorship of this series of books. This is good news. I hope that, in a small way, this book and its successors can act as a tribute to Professor

Kitwood's major contributions to the field of dementia care research.

Stephen Hopker
Bradford, March 1999

Chapter 1

Introduction

DRUG TREATMENTS AND THE PERSON WITH DEMENTIA

This book came about through the kind invitation of Professor Kitwood to set down some thoughts about the available evidence around drug treatments and dementia, as part of a series of guides intended to support clinicians and carers in their work with those affected by dementia. The book was originally going to address just the 'new' treatments in dementia, but in the end a wider approach was taken, to include drugs given for the psychiatric complications which can overlay and deepen the disabilities resulting from dementia. Some of these drugs have been in use for many years, and in recent times have been the subject of growing controversies – there is surprisingly little good quality evidence for the value of such medications. This guide will bring together some of the evidence of the effectiveness of these drug treatments and address the wider implications of their use.

Although the focus of this guide is the drug treatment of dementia-related problems, this does not mean that drugs are the first, only or best treatment for problems in persons with dementia: factors such as the approach of the carer and the care environment are arguably the largest factors in a patient's well-being. In my own experience, most practitioners in this field, including psychiatrists, see drug treatment for behavioural problems as being at most a small component of a person's total care needs, and only applicable for a minority of persons with dementia. In practice this does not mean that drug treatment should be used as a last resort (though it often is): I do want to stress that in many instances drug treatment has been too readily and too excessively prescribed, often with serious consequences for the recipients.

By contrast, good care (for people with any problems, not just dementia) takes a view of the whole person and often this enables carers to see more subtle and effective ways of coping than blunt sedation. By this I do not mean just a long list of tick-boxes to be checked off. Useful though such lists of assessments for memory problems, toileting needs, spiritual needs and so forth can be, there is a danger of missing the person themselves. Indeed, a great deal more could be said about the need to remember the *person* with dementia. This has been explored in greater depth and with more expertise by others (Kitwood 1997).

The kind of story below (although it is actually fictional) will be familiar to many who work with people who have dementia. When clinicians are asked to see a patient who is distressed – or distressing – there are strong expectations that they will 'do something', both by the clinician themselves, as well as the patient or carers. Clinicians tend to approach clients as patients, as someone who has an illness of some sort which must be identified and treated. Furthermore, clinicians usually suggest treatments which they are familiar with and can conveniently provide or arrange. Thus, the doctor in this example might have seen Emily as a case of dementia with some sort of behavioural disturbance, perhaps a psychosis secondary to her dementia – and so prescribed some tranquillizing, antipsychotic medication. The doctor would also have been aware of the staff's concerns regarding stress and risk to themselves, and possibly the impact of coping with Emily's problems upon their other residents (I have encountered such problems in the past, and responded similarly). At any rate, medication on this occasion proved to be worse than useless: fortunately the staff realised this and quite rightly took a professional decision to stop giving it and to explore other avenues. By no means all such problems can be resolved by such relatively simple measures, but many can.

Case Study

Emily was an eighty-two-year-old widow diagnosed with dementia in Alzheimer's disease of moderate severity. She also had arthritis. Her family doctor was called out because in the past few months she had been increasingly angry with care staff in the early mornings. A prescription of Melleril (thioridazine) the previous week had done nothing except cause some drowsiness and staff stopped it after a few doses. Conversations with staff revealed that the problem varied from day to day, with a pattern suggesting that when staff were very busy, the problem was worse. One of the senior carers undertook to look further and found that Emily became upset if she was rushed when dressing and more so if she was entirely dressed by carers (which was much quicker). Changes in her care plan to allow more time (she did not need a carer present continually) led to much of the verbal aggression disappearing.

DRUG TREATMENTS IN NURSING HOMES

The preceding views regarding the small and secondary importance of drug treatments for persons with dementia are not, I think, very contentious. Nonetheless, psychotropic drugs (i.e. drugs which are given to treat psychiatric problems) are widely prescribed to persons with dementia. Estimates of the numbers of nursing home residents who receive such medication range from 11 per cent to 74 per cent, with evidence from a recent community survey that the chance of receiving psychotropic drugs, especially antipsychotics, depends more on whether or not a person lives in an institution than whether or not they have dementia (Devanand and Levy 1995; Wills *et al.* 1997). Although persons admitted to residential or nursing care are more likely to be those with more problems, it is not clear that this is the only factor in the higher use of drug treatment. Indeed, this issue has occasionally aroused public debate – particularly, it would seem, in the US. In the rest of this introduction I look at this issue mostly from an American perspective, outlining the debate there and the legislation which resulted (Burke 1999, see below).

In the 1980s various studies were published which reflected concern about nursing homes and drug use. In one US study of a number of nursing homes it was found that the rates of antipsychotic drug treatment varied markedly from home to home (Ray, Federspiel and Schaffner 1980). Although the authors did not compare the patterns of diagnoses and problem behaviours between the homes, they did find that the rates of prescribing were strongly linked to the size of the homes and varied markedly between different physicians. Larger homes had higher treatment rates, and the greater the proportion of a home's residents under a single physician, the higher the prescribing rate of antipsychotics. The study did not collect data to tell us much about the cultures of care in these homes, but workers such as Kitwood and others (Kitwood and Bredin 1992) have done much work in describing the relationship between residents and professional carers, showing that particular homes can use generally positive, or adverse approaches. On the whole, the evidence from this field suggests that where homes are accommodating people with broadly the same set of needs, homes where residents are more likely to receive tranquillizing medications are also more likely to engage their residents in negative caring styles. So, to some degree, the extent of use of such drugs might act as a proxy for the quality of care in general.

Certainly, in the US, the issue of nursing home care and medication has continued to cause anxiety. For example, the title of one paper was *Drug Misuse in Nursing Homes: An Institutional Addiction?* (Waxman, Klein and Carner 1985). In it, the authors contended that not only was there evidence for excessive treatment of nursing home residents with psychiatric drugs, but that this over treatment originated in the institutions themselves – with hard pressed and untrained nursing aides being asked to take the brunt of care tasks. They pointed to the high turnover of such staff and suggested that, although the aides were at the bottom of a hierarchy, the institution owners needed to use them to deliver care at low financial costs. The authors suggested that demands by staff that their burden be eased led to the sedation of difficult residents through drug treatments. They suggested that if such patterns of drug treatment were withdrawn the homes could not cope – hence 'institutional' addiction.

Yet questions about unnecessary medication had been raised well before this time. In 1966 a paper from Colchester, England, related the author's doubts concerning the value of the use of chlorpromazine for elderly hospital in-patients who suffered from dementia, and concern that continuous medication use was often 'indiscriminate' (Barton and Hurst 1966). The study design would seem unusual nowadays but was not untypical then. All patients receiving chlorpromazine on six hospital wards were involved: after a week of observation, the chlorpromazine syrup on three wards was replaced by placebo (i.e. inactive) syrup. The study found that only about 20 per cent of patients who were switched to placebo showed a worsening of agitation and other problem behaviours. As an interesting sideline, the researchers asked each of the ward sisters to guess which medication was being given out – their responses did not differ significantly from random. Whatever one makes of the methods of this study now, the finding that for 80 per cent of recipients continued antipsychotics were at best useless (perhaps worse than useless for many) is a notable foreshadowing of similar conclusions made several decades later.

The concerns in the US over the excessive use of psychotropic drugs in homes, including references to 'chemical restraints' (Covert, Rodrigues and Solomon 1977), appear to have culminated in the Omnibus Budget Reconciliation Act legislation and accompanying regulations. Clinicians outside of the United States may be unfamiliar with OBRA-87, but this legislation and its accompanying guidelines have set out legal requirements regarding psychiatric drug treatments in US nursing homes – many of whose residents suffer from dementia.

OBRA-87 was followed by interpretative regulations for the Act (written by the Health Care Financing Administration) and the first set of these came into official effect in the autumn of 1990; there have been further regulations since. In essence, nursing homes will only receive healthcare reimbursement if the regulations concerning specified drug treatments are adhered to.

It would not be appropriate to describe these measures in detail, but in brief the OBRA-87 framework requires US nursing homes to ensure that medications covered by the Act are not prescribed unnecessarily, and that if prescribed they are regularly reviewed and where clinically possible, reduced with the aim of eventual withdrawal (Burke 1991). Antipsychotics were the first drug class to be subject to regulation (from 1990), followed by regulations for anti-anxiety and sedative drugs (in 1992). These later guidelines came in the wake of concerns over inappropriate replacement of antipsychotics by such medication (Borson and Doane 1997).

Having passed the legislation at national level, was there any impact on the ground? A survey of 39 nursing homes looked at the pre- and post-OBRA-87 prescribing rates of psychotropic medications (Borson and Doane 1997). The researchers found that whilst the prescribing rate of antipsychotics had fallen after the introduction of OBRA-87, the overall rates of psychotropic treatments stayed much the same, with higher rates of anti-anxiety treatments (in particular buspirone).

From the perspective of a British clinician, the very existence of legislation such as OBRA-87 is fairly remarkable and suggests that concerns in the US must have been high. There has been a study of prescribing practice in UK nursing homes which found that of the 24 per cent of residents receiving neuroleptics, only 12 per cent (approximately 1 in 8) had problems deemed under OBRA-87 to be suitable for such treatment (McGrath and Jackson 1997).

Is OBRA-87 an example which should followed, or an over reaction to problems which could have been addressed by other, less legalistic means? Certainly, OBRA-87 appears to carry a message that the welfare of nursing home residents is a matter for national concern – and it is interesting to note that, for whatever reasons, the issue has never achieved such a high profile in the UK. It is hoped that there will continue to be research into the impact of OBRA-87, in particular into how any drug treatment regulations affect the well-being of residents.

Chapter 2

Behavioural and Other Psychiatric Problems in Dementia

INTRODUCTION

Although memory and other cognitive problems are the central features of dementia, changes in behaviour and psychiatric symptoms such as disturbances of mood and perception are also very common. Up until recently, it was generally these observable problems which led to drug treatment in dementia. There is a tendency – exemplified by the literature quoted below – to focus on observable disturbances (i.e. 'problem behaviours'): this may run the risk of clinicians losing sight of the need to understand the personal experience of those affected by dementia, not least when attempting to weigh up the pros and cons of particular treatments (Kitwood and Bredin 1992; Kitwood 1997). Clinicians and others are also aware that behavioural and emotional difficulties do not arise in isolation and that there may be important triggers in the person's environment, to the extent that the 'problems' may largely lie in their environment, especially in how carers interact with the affected person. It is also important to consider the extent to which problems in dementia arise from the condition itself and how much a person's previous personality traits have a part to play: and indeed, as to whether persons with dementia undergo a change of personality (Hinchliffe, Katona and Livingston 1997).

OCCURRENCE OF PSYCHO-BEHAVIOURAL PROBLEMS IN DEMENTIA

Published surveys of behavioural and psychiatric problems in dementia tend to focus either on persons with clinically diagnosed Alzheimer's disease or to group people with any dementia sub-type together. Although there is some evidence of differences between dementia sub-types in terms of the relative *frequencies* of the occurrence of certain problems, they may occur to some extent in persons with any of the various forms of dementia.

Table 2.1 shows figures from a review of published papers on this topic (Tariot 1996). It gives the median (i.e. average or mid-point) of the range of the various reported frequencies of occurrence of problems and then the range itself (both shown as percentages of all patients). Individual patients may of course have more than one problem. I have re-ordered the list, by ranking the average (median) frequency with the most common problem being first.

It would appear from these figures that behaviours which are often seen as the most stressful or difficult, that is aggression and uncooperativeness, are in fact the least common at any one time, although up to 90 per cent of persons with dementia may have difficult behaviour at some time during their illness (Tariot 1996). By contrast, far and away the most frequent problem is withdrawal/passivity – which is little mentioned in the literature as a problem leading to drug treatment – unless identified with depression.

The large range of reported frequencies is somewhat striking:

Table 2.1 Frequency of Psycho-Behavioural Problems in Dementia

Problem	Median[1] (%)	Range[2] (%)
Withdrawn/passive	61	21–88
Agitation	44	10–90
Appetite disturbance	34	12.5–77
Delusions/other abnormal thoughts	33.5	10–73
Anxiety	31.8	0–50
Hallucinations	28	21–49
Sleep disturbance	27	0–47
Verbal aggression	24	11–51
Misperceptions (e.g. illusions)	23	1–49
Disturbed mood (usually depressed)	19	0–86
Physical aggression	14.3	0–46
Resistive/ uncooperative	14	27–65

Source: Tariot 1996

Tariot does not discuss this in his review, but in another paper it is suggested there is lack of consensus on how to assess non-cognitive problems and how to account for variations in the research settings. For example, rates of psychotic symptoms were lowest in dementia research centres, where patients with such

1   Median = middle value
2   Range = lowest and highest values

disturbances would be less likely to be referred and highest in surveys performed on acute hospital in-patients – who are often admitted precisely because of disturbed behaviour (Borson and Rishkind 1997).

The kinds of experiences labelled as 'psychotic' can be divided into two categories: abnormal perceptions (such as illusions and hallucinations) and abnormal beliefs (such as delusions). Hallucinations (false perceptions) are often of ordinary events, which may relate to personal memories, such as children coming into the house. Persons affected by dementia may also experience perceptual illusions, such as taking a change in floor covering to be a step. In terms of delusions (beliefs, usually false, held contrary to available evidence and out of keeping with that person's cultural norms) are often fairly straightforward, such as beliefs that theft has occurred or that neighbours want them to move out. Misidentification (e.g. of a child for a sibling) is quite common, as is the belief that the person is not living at their own home when they are (or that they are in their own home when in fact they are in hospital or residential care).

Many such delusions appear to be linked to the cognitive problems of dementia, such as disorientation in place or person, or misinterpretation of belongings mislaid by the person affected by dementia as stolen by others. Psychotic symptoms in dementia may only be evident for a few months and then only intermittently. There is some evidence that persons with dementia who suffer psychotic symptoms are likely to have more severe pathology and to decline more rapidly. There is some debate over whether antipsychotics may hasten decline, as these are often prescribed to persons with psychotic symptoms (McShane *et al.* 1997).

DISTRESSING PSYCHOTIC SYMPTOMS

People may experience psychotic symptoms which are not distressing and in such cases there seems little to recommend direct drug treatment. However, the following 'histories' illustrate some common psychotic symptoms that can affect people with dementia. For both people, these experiences were distressing and therefore merited intervention.

Case studies

David was a fifty-seven-year-old married man diagnosed with early onset dementia in Alzheimer's disease. At times he became physically aggressive towards his wife, telling her to get out of his home and demanding to know where his wife was. At such moments he called her Jane, the name of a sister. These delusions of misidentification persisted, medication having little impact. Respite through day care and regular stays in a residential home appeared to defer his eventual admission to permanent care.

Sarah was a seventy-year-old lady diagnosed with vascular type dementia. She frequently complained about intruders in the house and described them as a family with children who suddenly appeared in her front room, sitting on the settee but remaining silent. These distressing visual hallucinations were more or less stopped by a small dose of sulpiride (an antipsychotic medication).

MOOD PROBLEMS

Turning to mood problems, there may be questions as to whether 'depression' in a person with dementia is comparable to the 'depression' seen in persons with classical depressive disorder. Certainly persons with dementia may have a full depressive syndrome as well, but frequently only some features of depression can be identified, such as poor sleep, or tearfulness, or withdrawal. It is often difficult to distinguish such symptoms from dementia. The figures from research into depressive problems and dementia would bear out such difficulties; the range of estimates for prevalence for 'depression' being 0 per cent to 86 per cent, with a range of 5–15 per cent for the more tightly defined major depression (Borson and Rishkind 1997).

AGITATION AND AGGRESSION

Another area of debate concerns the meaning of such terms as 'agitation' and 'aggression'. 'Aggression' is widely used term, sometimes including verbal aggression, but at others confined to physical aggression. Patel and Hope have offered a more specific definition: 'Aggressive behaviour is an *overt* act, involving the delivery of *noxious* stimuli to (but not necessarily aimed at) another object, or self, which is clearly *not accidental*' (Patel and Hope 1993 p.458). In another paper aggression is approached as one part of a wider agitation syndrome: this approach is based on a review of literature and a study (Cohen-Mansfield and Billig 1986). The authors suggest that for a behaviour to be considered as agitation for the purposes of study and treatment in its own right, it must be observable, not linked to other factors (e.g. sleep disturbance) and not an action which could be otherwise explained (thus, a purposeful walk, even if the person ended up getting lost, would be excluded). Cohen-Mansfield and Billig suggest that agitation is a cluster of various behaviours which can be grouped from two approaches (or 'dimensions'), namely verbal/non-verbal, and aggressive/non-aggressive. This is summarized in table 2.2 below.

In recent years, studies of treatments for agitation or aggression have often used assessment instruments which aim to define such behaviours, but other studies do not appear to have used such approaches, which makes it harder to apply their findings clinically – because if it is unclear what behaviour is referred to in a report then it is not clear whether this is the same behaviour the clinician has identified in other situations. Many authors advocate that dementia-related problems are assessed systematically, which requires clinicians to be as careful, thorough and objective as possible in describing a person's problems.

Table 2.2 A Classification of Agitation		
	Aggressive	Non-aggressive
Verbal	curses, threats	strange noises, screaming, repetitious pleas for help, meaningless repetition/ talk
Non-verbal	hitting, fighting, grabbing, hurting oneself, deliberate falls	pacing, wandering aimlessly
Source: Cohen-Mansfield and Billig 1986		

CONCLUSIONS

It is possible to attempt to generate a coordinated idea of the various psychiatric (e.g. perceptual, emotional and behavioural) problems a person with dementia may have by diagnosing a psychiatric syndrome which is deemed to be secondary to the dementia: this 'psychobehavioral metaphor' can guide treatment, for example by indicating antipsychotics for people with psychotic symptoms (Tariot, Schneider and Katz 1995). Although such treatment by resemblance has a logical appeal, the biological rationale for it is unclear – and as will be seen, the treatment evidence would not suggest such 'syndromes' in dementia are comparable in terms of responsiveness.

Overall, such observational or medical approaches focus on the outward behaviours of a patient with little reference to their inner experiences. This does make for easier observation, but a literature has emerged on the experience of patients and the patterns of interactions between people with dementia and their carers (Kitwood and Bredin 1992), which leads on naturally to the concept of person-centred care – that is, an approach to the understanding of someone as a *whole person*. This approach seeks to begin from that person's position – from the 'inside out' – rather than objectifying (depersonalizing) them through descriptions which are little more than lists of problems or disorders. There are also strong indications that the behaviour of persons affected by dementia is not simply the result of individual characteristics, but is instead a product of that person's potential repertoire of behaviours and their environment, perhaps most critically the quality of their relationships and interactions with others.

Chapter 3

Principles of Drug Treatment in Dementia

ASSESSING SUITABILITY FOR TREATMENT

When considering drug treatment for someone with dementia, assessment is required to answer a number of questions, which are explored below.

In what ways and to what extent could treatment be expected to help this person?

It is important for all parties involved in the care of a person with dementia to be clear as to why drug treatment is being considered. The first and usually only reason is to enhance that person's overall well-being: other reasons, such as the safety of other persons should only be considered *in extremis* and usually as a temporary measure, pending more satisfactory care arrangements. 'Overall well-being' is a key phrase to note: it means that a person's quality of life, taken as a whole, is enhanced by treatment. This is a somewhat difficult dimension to measure, yet clinicians will be familiar with situations where particular problems (such as agitation) are reduced, although sometimes at the cost of new problems (such as sedation). It is a further challenge to attempt such an appraisal from the patient's point of view, yet this is the only meaningful interpretation of 'well-being'. Within this framework, clinicians, alongside carers, should identify problem areas which need to be tackled. In setting out such objectives for treatment, clinicians should be cautious of being restricted by limitations imposed by the care setting (e.g. staffing levels), unless there are compelling reasons for retaining such constraints.

Which particular treatments could be of benefit to this person with dementia?

Clinicians should consider the full range of potentially effective interventions applicable to the person's identified problems, in order to check that there are not alternative actions which could be taken.

Case study

Florence was a seventy-four-year-old lady affected by dementia, to the extent that she relied on her husband for prompting and guidance about many daily tasks, although she still shopped and cooked for herself. She took his sudden death 'well', in that she did not become highly distressed, but over the following weeks her neighbours became increasingly concerned about her forgetfulness. They contacted her son, who lived over a hundred miles away, who visited and found her to be very quiet and to have lost weight. He arranged for her to be admitted to a residential home, but she became very unsettled and slightly confused. This led to a brief hospital admission after which she was discharged back to her own home and for over a year coped well on a practical level with regular community care support. She appeared to benefit from attending a therapeutic day hospital, in particular from a depression support group and one-to-one work with a nurse therapist. Eventually she became too forgetful to participate in more formal therapy groups, but still enjoyed social contact from other activities.

This illustrative history covers several points, including the way depression and increased confusion are often triggered by loss (first of her husband, then of her home and independence) and how a variety of inputs (practical support, social contact, therapy groups) can combine to good effect. Finally, the needs of people with dementia tend to change with time, so interventions need to be kept under continual review.

Are current treatments helping or hindering this person?

Current interventions, including medication, should be reviewed, as many drugs are capable of exacerbating confusion (e.g. antipsychotics, minor tranquillizers, antidepressants and anti-parkinsonian medications). Similar considerations apply to agitation or aggression – even drugs which were prescribed to alleviate such problems may paradoxically worsen them. Again, in assessing withdrawal or depressive-style problems, drugs such as sedatives may require review before any new drugs are prescribed.

Would a particular treatment be safe for this person?

In following the ancient (Hippocratic) injunction to 'do no harm', prior to prescribing any new medication there should always be a thorough consideration of any risks of harm through treatment. Thus, advanced age, low body weight or general frailty would all indicate the need for caution. The presence of certain medical conditions, or the risk of interaction with other medications may also limit the range of safe options.

Case study

Sarah was a seventy-six-year-old widow (eventually) diagnosed as being affected by severe dementia in Lewy-body disease. She had recently moved from a residential home to a nursing home nearer to her family, but staff reported severe agitation (i.e. great distress and restlessness, leading to exhaustion). She had become drowsy and unsteady on even the smallest dose of haloperidol (an antipsychotic). Subsequent changes in medication found she could not tolerate low doses of sulpiride (a newer antipsychotic drug). Trazodone, an antidepressant sometimes used for agitation, was ineffective. The only medication which made any useful difference to her distress was a low dose of lorazepam (a minor tranquillizer). Meanwhile, she had spent some time in hospital and then made a failed return to the first home. After a return to hospital a move to a specialist nursing home resulted in a period of one-to-one assessment and care and her levels of agitation gradually lessened.

Such odysseys are not uncommon: eventually, a home was found which offered an intensive approach over the long term and this almost entirely removed the need for medication.

Will the drug be taken by this person?

Clinicians also need to consider factors in drug concordance, such as a person's views about medication. Memory impairment (especially in conjunction with multiple drug regimes) is a problem in the case of people who live alone, and may rule out some drug treatments altogether or at least require simplified prescriptions. It may be possible for all medication to be taken at one time to facilitate remembering, or for it to be given by a visiting carer. The use of 'dosette boxes' may be of value – these being trays with a week's medication already set out in slots for each time of day. Obviously this system would not work with people with more severe impairment. Other practical problems may include visual impairment, arthritis affecting finger joints and swallowing difficulties.

SOME ETHICAL ISSUES

If, after assessment, the prescribing clinician has identified a medication as potentially of sufficient benefit for the target problems, safe and likely to be taken, then treatment should be offered. The patient should be given as much information as they can absorb regarding the reasons for offering treatment. People with dementia often have reduced scope for consent and medication should be discussed with their families or advocates. There is an issue here of how a person with dementia is viewed, for example, in their capacity for choice, and indeed their personhood. Sometimes clinicians – and carers – can act as if the person concerned had no scope to make choices, or can even treat the person with dementia as if, because the ability to *express* wishes or inner experience was much diminished, that person therefore had little in the way of thoughts or desires. Close attendance to a person's utterances or observation of his or her gestures and responses can often identify a person's wishes.

Quite clearly, however, there will be situations where even if a person's views can be ascertained, the severity of their impairment does preclude informed decisions about issues such as care settings or treatments (be they medical or psychological). Many countries have passed mental health legislation which, under circumstances of high risk, allows the treatment of persons without their consent – but this does not reduce the need to offer such information.

BEGINNING TREATMENT

Assuming medication has been accepted or legally permitted, it should be commenced, usually at doses well below the usual range for fit – or younger – adults. In ordinary practice doses should 'start low and rise slow', perhaps no more than at weekly intervals, and in most cases should never even approach the typical levels used in other conditions: so, for example, the doses of antipyschotics given to persons affected by dementia should normally be much lower than those used in schizophrenia.

There are three main reasons for such caution in prescribing, which are outlined below.

1: Age-related changes in drug absorption and distribution

The way in which a drug moves through a person's system (the 'pharmacodynamics') is often different in persons who are aged and therefore in many of the people with dementia (I am unaware of data about younger people with dementia in respect of this issue). In general, these changes mean that lower doses are more suitable: they are safer and often sufficient. Whilst drug absorption is usually not much altered, for some drugs, such as benzodiazepines, it is slowed down. Absorption may also be slowed by other drugs which reduce the rate of stomach emptying (such as anticholinergic drugs). A slower absorption rate may result in the drug having a slower onset of action and also a more prolonged effect.

After absorption, a drug is distributed throughout the body – indeed, only a tiny proportion reaches the brain. One influence on drug distribution is the extent to which the drug is bound to proteins in the blood (this makes it unavailable to act). There is evidence that this factor is less important than the extent of distribution to fatty tissues – where many psychoactive drugs are highly absorbed (Pollock and Mulsant 1995). Such fatty tissue acts as a reservoir for the drug, tending to slow the onset and the cessation of action. Although older persons may, on the whole, have a lower body weight, they tend to have a greater proportion of fat: so this is another factor leading to drugs in older persons having a more gradual onset of action – but also a more prolonged one.

Most drugs are subject to metabolism, that is, to being broken down (through biological catalysts, i.e. metabolic enzymes). This will ultimately result in the production of chemicals which are inactive, or which can more easily be eliminated from the body. There is evidence that the activity of some, but not all, metabolic enzymes reduces in older age. Furthermore, a great deal of metabolism takes place in the liver, the blood circulation of which diminishes with age. Thus, the rate of liver metabolism is often slowed, which is of particular significance with drugs which are normally highly metabolized in the liver before reaching the general circulation. The overall effect of age-related changes in drug metabolism in many drugs is to slow their rate of deactivation and eventual removal from the body.

There is a further important aspect of drug metabolism, in respect to drug interactions. Drugs may alter the activity levels of the metabolic enzymes themselves – either to increase their activity ('enzyme induction') or to diminish it ('enzyme inhibition'). Since the same enzyme may metabolize many drugs, this can have significant effects on the blood levels and length of action of other drugs. This is addressed further in the section on drug interactions.

After drugs have been absorbed, distributed and (usually) metabolized within the body, they – or their metabolites – are removed (elimination). For the most part, this takes place through the kidneys. Once again, research in older persons finds an age-related decline in the efficiency of these organs, so drugs or active metabolites which are eliminated through the kidneys may have reduced rates of clearance from the body.

Much of the above information is based upon measurements of drug levels within the blood, and a convention has been developed to summarize the net effects of all the above processes, namely measurement of the time it takes for blood levels to fall to half their value from their peak, after one dose has been given. This time is called the 'half-life'. Research shows that the time taken for drug levels to stabilize by reaching a 'steady state' is in proportion to the half-life. It should be noted that drugs may have a more prolonged effect than their half-life would suggest.

As should be clear by now, for the most part these age-related changes in pharmacodynamics point in a similar direction: that the dosage required to reach a particular blood level in the elderly is usually less than in younger people and that the effects of the drug will be relatively prolonged.

2: Altered drug actions

The second reason to be cautious in drug treatment in dementia concerns the actions of a drug itself. As with the above discussion of pharmacodynamics, much research is focused on older adults rather than persons of any age with dementia: despite the problems this raises in some respects for treating younger persons with dementia, the overall indications regarding older persons are that drug side effects may become more troublesome.

In some cases there appears to be an age-related risk of side effects due to changes in other bodily systems. For example, a reduction in the mechanisms to maintain blood pressure on standing leads to an increased risk of dizziness or falls. At other times, co-existent conditions may increase risks: for example, persons with heart disease may be more prone to disorders of the heart beat, or effects on the eyes may increase the risk of worsening unrecognized or untreated glaucoma. Mobility problems will clearly combine adversely with side effects such as muscle weakness. Dopamine blocking drugs (such as antipsychotics) may worsen pre-existing Parkinson's disease.

There appears to be an increased risk of such drugs causing long-term, or even permanent side effects such as tardive dyskinesia (a kind of movement disorder described later). Finally, persons with dementia are more prone to epilepsy, and a number of drugs can also increase this risk.

3: Drug interactions

Drug interactions are of course important constraints on prescribing for any patient, but tend to be more of an issue for persons affected by dementia for several reasons:

- people with dementia are often elderly and so more prone to other conditions and therefore more likely to be taking other medication

- their underlying brain pathology may be associated with other conditions requiring treatment (e.g. vascular dementia associated with heart disease)

- difficulties in relieving the psychological or behavioural problems of dementia may lead to agents being added one to another, rather than tried one at a time

- drug treatment for dementia problems may produce side effects which lead to the need for other treatments (e.g. antipsychotic medication causing Parkinsonism, leading to treatment with anticholinergics such as procyclidine).

Drug interactions may arise in various ways, essentially relating to the above mentioned stages of absorption, distribution, metabolism, elimination and drug action.

Examples of interactions with absorption have been given already. A frequently mentioned interaction concerning distribution is that between warfarin and other drugs which tend to bind to blood protein. Because warfarin is highly bound to blood protein it tends to displace other drugs, so raising their unbound ('free') drug levels. Thus, if a patient already on a drug is given warfarin, the free levels of the first drug may rise, perhaps causing side effects; conversely, if a patient has been on a drug and warfarin together and warfarin is then stopped, the free levels of the other drug will fall as more of it becomes bound to the blood proteins.

There is a growing understanding of drug interactions through alterations of metabolism. For example, antipsychotics such as haloperidol or thioridazine tend to inhibit a particular metabolic enzyme; as this enzyme also metabolizes other drugs such as antidepressants there is the possibility of antidepressant levels being higher than if no antipsychotic had been prescribed. Interactions through drug metabolism may also have the opposite effect of enzyme induction. For example, certain anti-epilepsy drugs may increase the activity of enzymes metabolizing some antidepressants, causing blood levels to fall below what would be normal for the prescribed dose, so the anti-depressant may not work so well.

Regarding drug action, there are again many examples of how the action of one drug affects that of another. Thus, antipsychotics may diminish the effect of treatments for Parkinson's disease through opposing actions on dopamine. On the other hand, the effects of re-uptake inhibiting anti-depressants may add to those of other antidepressants which inhibit neurotransmitter metabolism and so increase the risk of adverse events.

REVIEWING AND DISCONTINUING TREATMENT

Prescribing for behavioural or psychiatric symptoms in dementia should be seen as a trial of treatment and if successful, a temporary measure. Whatever factors led to the original disturbed behaviour may well abate. Failure to improve is another common reason to review drug treatment; another assessment may be required and other treatment options considered. One simple option would be to increase the drug dosage, if that is safely possible; another, of course, would be to discontinue the drug and check if the original problem still merited drug treatment.

Having established that a particular drug is of overall benefit, its continued value should be monitored. For example, there is evidence that drugs such as antipsychotics might be withdrawn after a few months without causing problems in most persons with dementia (Bridges-Parlet, Knopman and Steffes 1997). Generally speaking, drugs given for psychiatric or behavioural problems in dementia should be not be given for more than a few months. The research evidence on antipsychotic medication suggests that in most persons these drugs could be discontinued without difficulty. Cognitive enhancing drugs, if deemed to be of overall value, are likely to be prescribed in the long term (how long is not yet clear), but even these might eventually be judged of no value in someone who has deteriorated to profound dementia. Minor tranquillizers such as benzodiazepines (e.g. temazepam) should not normally be given on a regular basis for more than a month or so because of the risk of the development of dependency.

On the whole, when a drug is to be discontinued this should be done gradually. Sometimes trial reductions in medication lead to a deterioration, and restitution of the original dose is followed by an improvement: the obvious course would then be to continue the medication for a while longer, although this would not mean the medication should be continued indefinitely. In some circumstances there are reasons, after proper review, to continue drug treatment in the longer term. This would include drugs given for pre-existing conditions such as schizophrenia, or recurrent mood disorders.

Jenny's experience, described below, illustrates how an emphasis on assessing particular outcomes might miss the overall impact of treatment – which, it should be stated in the case of drugs like donepezil, offers only a temporary improvement and does not halt the underlying progression of the dementia. Quite clearly, improvement in cognition and daily living skills could well enhance overall quality of life, but it is the latter which is the final arbiter of the value of treatment, however difficult it may be to define and measure.

Case study

Jenny was well adjusted to the routine in her nursing home. She was in a relatively benign emotional state and seemed to be enjoying the art and music programs in which she actively participated. After beginning Aricept (donepezil), Jenny regained insight into her situation. For example, she remembered that she did not want to be in a nursing home, and insisted that she be allowed to leave. She also refused to participate in any support programs because the participants were 'too slow'. (Post 1998)

BRAIN PATHOLOGY, CHEMISTRY AND DRUG ACTIONS IN DEMENTIA
Brain pathology

There appear to be three main types of brain pathology which are associated with dementia. About fifty per cent of persons diagnosed with dementia syndrome are thought to have Alzheimer's disease. Clinicians will also be familiar with vascular dementia where blood vessels have abnormalities or there have been a number of small strokes. This is present in twenty to thirty per cent of persons with dementia. Dementia in vascular brain disease is associated with vascular problems elsewhere in the body, such as heart disease or hypertension. Perhaps ten per cent of persons with dementia have both Alzheimer's and vascular type brain disease.

In more recent years a third type of pathology, 'diffuse Lewy-body disease', has been recognised; here, abnormalities (Lewy-bodies) seen in neurones within one small part of the brain in Parkinson's disease are found more widely, and associated with a dementia in which there is an increased likelihood of fluctuation in severity, hallucinations and movement problems – the latter resembling Parkinson's disease. Of particular relevance to drug treatments, persons with this form of dementia are more prone to severe side effects from antipsychotic medication. Diffuse Lewy-body disease may be present in around 15 per cent of persons with dementia (Esiri 1991).

Moving away from specific pathologies, there is a growing body of evidence about the damage to brain tissue which seems to occur in several forms of dementia. It appears that apart from the specific types of pathology, there are other processes, such as excessive and damaging inflammatory reactions. This suggests that whilst direct treatment of some pathologies may be difficult, reducing some of the associated abnormal reactions of brain tissue may well be possible. In the case of vascular dementias, it may be possible to reduce brain tissue damage in the first place, by reducing the risk of impaired blood flow.

Brain chemistry

There has in recent decades been an explosion of knowledge about chemical processes within the brain and this has enabled a massive research effort in this area in respect of dementia. This research is mostly focused upon Alzheimer's disease – there is much less reference to abnormal brain chemistry in other types of dementia pathology.

According to current thinking, the key element in brain function is the activity of nerve cells, or neurones. Neurones are electrically active cells, and signals are passed between them by means of chemicals called neurotransmitters. When a neurone 'fires' an electrical discharge, a wave of electrical activity moves down a long nerve fibre and causes a small amount of neurotransmitter to be released. This happens very close to another neurone. The neurotransmitter then links to, or 'binds' a particular site (the receptor) on the second neurone. This receptor binding leads to further changes which typically alter the second neurone's electrical status. In order to avoid 'jamming' the signals, the binding neurotransmitter must be removed quickly. This may happen through its being broken down (metabolized) or taken up again into the neurone which released it ('re-uptake').

Drug actions

Drugs can affect this chemical signalling process in many different ways. For example, the amount of transmitter available for release can be increased by providing more of the chemicals needed to produce it; or the rate at which the released transmitter is taken up again or metabolized can be altered (e.g. re-uptake inhibition). It is also possible to de-activate the receptor sites; for example, by occupying (blocking) them with chemicals that take a long time to move off the receptors and so cutting down the signals that can pass through.

Some neurotransmitters operate in a general way and are not messengers of specific information (such as the perception of a sensation, or the generation of a particular movement). Instead, they regulate activity by other neurones. All of the drugs used in dementia appear to affect such generalized, 'tone-setting' functions.

It should be stressed that there are many other chemicals thought to act as neurotransmitters, that there are thousands of interconnections between individual neurones and that there are many different ways in which such connections function, beyond the highly simplified description just given. In other words, although much knowledge has been gained in recent years about brain function, much more remains to be learnt, both in terms of normal function as well as the various forms of dementia pathology.

Specific neurotransmitters: Acetylcholine

The cognitive deficits in dementia have for a long time been linked to deficiencies in a neurotransmitter called acetylcholine. Outside the brain this chemical has a role in the autonomic nervous system (i.e. the part of the nervous system which lies beyond conscious control) which regulates the functions of various organs, such as the heart, bowels, bladder and the eyes – so drugs affecting acetylcholine often have side effects related to the functioning of those organs. Within the brain, however, it has been found that blocking acetylcholine receptors impairs memory. Boosting acetylcholine levels, however, by inhibiting a chemical which enables the breakdown of acetylcholine (called acetylcholinesterase) will tend to reverse such problems. The brain structures associated with acetylcholine are found to be damaged in Alzheimer's disease.

Despite the strong evidence linking this neurotransmitter to the cognitive problems in Alzheimer's disease, it may be that acetylcholine disorder is related to other problems (e.g. delusions, agitation or apathy) and also that other neuro-transmitter abnormalities may be involved in cognitive problems (Cummings and Kaufer 1996). Thus, drugs that boost acetylcholine might treat some dementia-related problems, but at the same time be unable to combat all aspects of the memory and other skills impairments upon which such drugs are explicitly targeted.

Other neurotransmitters

There is evidence for reduced activity levels of *serotonin*, or 5–HT (5–hydroxy-tryptamine) and *noradrenaline* in persons with dementia. Deficiencies of these neurotransmitters are also implicated in persons without dementia in problems such as low mood and aggression. There may be links between abnormalities in 5–HT and specific behavioural problems in persons with dementia, but the picture is by no means clear or complete.

Chapter 4

Looking at Evidence

ADVANTAGES AND LIMITATIONS OF EVIDENCE-BASED PRACTICE

This guide claims to be based, as far as is possible, upon some of the available published research. Some may question such an approach, believing that clinical experience is of more relevance to everyday practice than academic research. Whilst this is true in that research settings and study participants are not, almost by definition, identical to those in routine care, there are nonetheless compelling reasons – outlined later on – to distrust one's own experience as a sufficient source of information. However, this guide is indeed 'based upon' evidence: whatever the quality of evidence about treatments, this still needs to be sensitively applied in a given situation to a particular person. Good quality evidence supports the task of clinical judgement – it does not supplant it. Indeed, there are times when a clinician may need to step back from the often hidden assumptions that underlie research in order to consider fresh approaches: thus, much drug-related research seems to imply that brain pathology is the sole factor in dementia, and some observational studies seem to focus on outward behaviour and all but ignore the person's own thoughts and feelings.

EFFICACY AND EFFECTIVENESS

Readers of reports about clinical trials are likely to come across the term *efficacy* and possibly *effectiveness*. Efficacy refers to how well a treatment works when studied in a clinical trial; effectiveness is how well the treatment works in clinical practice. Most of the trial data in this book is around efficacy, which means caution must be exercised in applying the research findings to particular settings. This is because of evidence that (in other fields of psychiatry) the efficacy reported in highly formalized trials is not matched by effectiveness in general clinical usage (Guscott and Taylor 1994).

STUDY DESIGN

Some of the earlier published data on drug treatments in dementia are simple 'case series', or even individual reports, describing the response to a particular drug in one or more patients. Recollections of particular patients may be useful – indeed, these constitute 'clinical experience', but there is a danger that case studies of patients who responded very well (or very badly) are more likely to be published than those – usually the majority – who show less extreme responses to treatment. This bias toward extreme outcomes may also apply when clinicians recall and share their experiences. There are other problems with only using ordinary clinical experience as a guide to practice, as outlined below.

Evidence from treatment trials suggests that if patients are given some form of treatment – even a dummy treatment (placebo) then a certain proportion will improve: this may happen in ordinary clinical practice, as well as in research trials (and is another reason to be cautious about relying just on clinical experience). This placebo response may be due to a number of factors, such as:

- the person with dementia benefits from the increased attention and contact resulting from being in a trial

- there has been spontaneous improvement of the condition (some conditions will improve without specific treatment)

- the condition shows variable severity (in a fluctuating disorder, some patients will appear to have improved within a given time period simply because their condition was, by chance, worse at the time of initial assessment than at outcome assessment)

- there could be a 'practice effect' (where performance might improve through repetition rather than treatment)

- people's (the patient's, carers' or clinicians') expectations of the response could affect the outcome through hope that a new treatment may work better than previous treatments, or better than no treatment at all.

Because of such problems, researchers often move on from the case series approach and use a control group design. The idea is to 'control' or allow for non-drug factors within the study treatment outcome by giving a different treatment to a comparable group of patients. Normally patients should be allocated to one or other group by chance – the trial is randomized.

Where the kind of treatment being given is known to all parties, the study is termed 'open'. Unfortunately, this does not eliminate undue expectations of response – and may increase the risk of participants being treated unequally in other ways. Therefore, researchers have devised studies with blinding – where participants are 'blind' to the kind of treatment given. Where the treatment is unknown only by patients the study is 'single blind': where no participant (patient, carer, clinician or assessor) knows the treatment, the study is 'double-blind'.

Putting the above aspects of clinical trial design together, it is often held that the best drug trials will be randomized, double-blind and placebo controlled: there are some grounds to question this model as the universal 'gold standard' – some of which I have listed below. It should be noted that there are many other significant aspects of trial design which are addressed by specialist texts on research methods.

It is also important, when looking through published literature, to be aware of a problem stemming from the medium itself, namely publication bias. Trials where a positive response occurred are more likely to be published than other instances where improvement was uncertain or absent. This applies to all forms of treatment reports – case series as well as larger controlled trials. Publication bias may affect reviews (and meta-analyses, where data from several studies is pooled) in that if some treatment trials have been omitted from the literature there is a risk of drawing the wrong conclusions when bringing together the findings of the reviewed papers.

LIMITATIONS OF CONTROLLED TRIALS

The above points indicate that carefully conducted double- blind controlled trials (especially placebo controlled) are a useful way to answer questions about a drug's clinical value. Such trials do have limitations, however:

- Trials often study highly selected populations. They look for people with clear-cut diagnoses and a relative absence of other health problems and other medications. They also only study those referred by clinicians and for whom consent is obtained. Not all clinicians, carers or patients may wish to subject themselves or others to treatment allocated on a random basis, when one of the possible treatments is a placebo or of unclear value (Devanand and Levy 1995).

- It is well recognized that blinding may fail – for example, a treatment may have clearly recognisable side effects.

- Some interventions cannot be blinded at all – for example direct care approaches or occupational therapies, so trial evidence may be seen as of lesser quality, leading to an undue priority being given to treatments which can be tested by double-blind trials.

- Not all important issues around psychological or behavioural problems may be readily amenable to measurement, which may mean there are important outcomes which are less easily measured – such as patient quality of life – which are given less consideration in the appraisal of a treatment's value.

- Essential components of the nature and treatment of the disorder such as environmental factors, may be omitted from consideration.

Despite these significant concerns, the randomized double-blind trial is recognized and funded as a powerful tool in assessing the efficacy of drug treatments. So for the time being – and in this book – such trials will be the main source of evidence on drug treatment.

INTERPRETING THE RESULTS OF A TRIAL

The results of a trial are usually reported in a number of ways – for example, mean scores on a rating scale, or associations between potential factors and outcome. Response rates (the proportions of persons in each treatment group who have certain outcomes) are relatively easy to understand and apply in clinical situations. The difference between different peoples' responses to treatments is the relative treatment effect.

For example, suppose a particular treatment was compared to placebo medication in a trial setting: 55 per cent of patients given the test treatment improved, as compared to 35 per cent of patients given the control treatment – i.e. placebo. This would indicate a treatment effect of 20 per cent, meaning that for every 100 patients given a treatment, there would be 20 more patients on active treatment deriving some benefit than those taking placebo. The chances of one patient benefiting will be 20/100, i.e. one in five. From the clinicians' point of view five people on average would need to be treated for one to obtain benefit. This last figure is referred to as the Number Needed to Treat (or NNT).

These figures are based upon the particular patients involved in a study. When it comes to applying those results to other patients there will be some uncertainty about whether the results are 'real'. For example, suppose a study comparing two treatments found that 20 per cent more people were likely to improve with a particular treatment: how sure could you be that this treatment really was 20 per cent better? Confidence that there was a real difference between treatments would be less if the difference was small: on the other hand, it would be greater if the effect was seen in more people.

One way to express the extent of confidence in a result is to calculate a confidence interval, which is the range within which you predict the 'real' value lies, with a given level of confidence. Typically these are reported at a 95 per cent level of confidence (i.e. a 95% confidence that the true value lies within the quoted range). When looking at the difference between treatments, if the lower limit of the 95 per cent confidential interval reaches or falls below zero, this means that one cannot say with 95 per cent confidence that there is any real difference: the same applies when comparing two figures and the CI of one overlaps the CI of the other. When differences fail to reach the target level of confidence, this is usually referred to as a 'non-significant' difference.

Another aspect of confidence intervals is that they project a range of 'true' figures (as suggested by the data). The point is that although the 'true' figure is most likely around the actual average or proportion measured, the intervals indicate the 'bounds of possibility' – so the 'true' figure might be a good deal higher or lower than at first seems. Often the 'true' figure becomes clearer after several studies have been reported. For example, the earlier reports of a definite treatment effect with tacrine (a putative cognitive enhancing agent), have not been borne out by a subsequent meta-analysis.

Clinicians should be wary of the term 'significant'. A difference in some measure in a particular group of patients may indeed be *statistically* significant, but the practical or clinical significance is a different matter. For example, with a large enough sample it may be possible to show that a particular treatment is 'significantly' better than placebo according to a particular scale – but if the actual difference is very small, clinicians and others may question the value such a small difference would have to individuals. There have been debates around such issues in relation to some of the new dementia treatments.

The presence or absence of statistical significance usually leads researchers to draw conclusions about the value of the study treatment. Of course, even if the statistics indicate a particular conclusion, this still might be wrong. There are two broad categories of errors which can be made in such research. First, drawing the false conclusion that there is a difference between two treatments, when there is not: this is often called a 'Type I error'. The second is to conclude that there is no difference when there is – a 'Type II error'.

Type I errors may lead to new treatments being given in the mistaken belief that they are effective, or more effective than other treatments. Type II errors may lead to potentially effective or superior treatments being rejected. These errors apply in other areas too – for example, in estimating the comparative risks attending various treatments. In this instance, a Type II error could mean that a treatment which is actually more hazardous is given under the false impression that it is as safe as other treatments. One common reason for the occurrence of Type II errors is studying too few patients: as the discussion regarding confidence intervals explained, smaller numbers of subjects are linked to more uncertainty about outcome and so statistical significance is harder to achieve.

Another point which clinicians will be aware of is the question of how readily conclusions about treating *groups* of people will apply to the *individual*. Quite often, average response rates are reported (e.g. changes in mean scores) and one might think that such an average change occurred for all subjects – yet individuals respond very differently, both in terms of therapeutic gains and adverse events. This means that, irrespective of how well established a drug treatment may be in general, every particular occasion of its use should be looked upon as a treatment trial for that individual.

Returning to the interpretation of trial results, it is often the case that a number of the patients originally in the trial fail to remain for the duration of the study. Such discontinuations, or 'drop-outs' may occur for any reason, but are often the result of adverse events (which may or may not be linked to treatment) and failure to improve. In trials concerning dementia this may be a more complex issue than usual, since along with the expectations of patients and clinicians, relatives also make a significant contribution in terms of reporting positive and adverse outcomes, and indeed in consenting to the person with dementia remaining in the trial. Bearing in mind such limitations, discontinuation rates due to adverse events can give some indication of tolerance, especially when compared to placebo drop-out rates.

Concerning response rates and other analyses of outcome, it is better for these to be reported for all persons commencing the treatment (called 'intent-to-treat' analysis) since only including those who completed the trial may bias the results. For example, if patients who do not improve left a study early, analyses based just on those completing the trial could be selective for those who benefited. Again, if the drug takes some time to show benefit, analyses which exclude patients who dropped out early will tend to show a more optimistic treatment effect than those including everyone who commenced treatment. Since clinicians will want to give advice about treatments before commencing them, the more inclusive (intent-to-treat) figures will be more helpful than response rates based on a narrower set of patients.

HOW GOOD IS THE EVIDENCE?

If the drug treatments in dementia were overwhelmingly effective and safe, then perhaps such 'academic' issues as addressed above would not be of concern to front-line clinicians. But such treatments are not so obviously effective, in terms of the measures used or their overall impact; and a number of them are not obviously safe, either. It is surprising that, considering the widespread and large scale use of various medications, the total evidence base for all drug treatments in dementia is somewhat small. Much of current practice seems to date from early clinical impressions and published data from open trials or case reports. Reviewers have noted that such studies tend to over-estimate the efficacy of treatments – that is, they suggest an apparent level of efficacy which is not replicated in a double-blind controlled study. One factor is the relatively high placebo response to many drug treatments in dementia – perhaps suggestive of the strong but non drug related effects of care and attention. This indicates caution in the routine use of treatments which clinical experience or case reports suggest may be 'promising' but which remain untested in an adequate trial, and where 'efficacy' may derive from fairly specific and possibly narrow criteria which do not take into account the overall impact of a drug upon a person's well-being.

Chapter 5

The New Treatments for Dementia

A few years ago a book such as this would have hardly mentioned drugs like cognitive enhancers or other possible dementia treatments, let alone set aside a chapter on the subject. Yet now, in the late 1990s, few people involved with the care and treatment of persons with dementia will be unaware of the developments in this area, and of the controversies surrounding them. One of these controversies – at least in the UK – has been about whether the small (average) advantage they may offer justifies their cost.

In the first part of this chapter, evidence about drugs intended to enhance cognitive performance in people with dementia is reviewed. Such treatments do not address the pathological processes causing damage to neurones. Later in this chapter there is some information about other drugs – some new, others older drugs which have not been used in dementia – which may prevent neuronal damage.

COGNITIVE ENHANCING AGENTS

Cognitive enhancers are given with the intention of improving cognitive performance on a symptomatic basis: they do so by addressing one of the neurotransmitter defects in dementia, that is, the relative lack of acetylcholine. Being symptomatic treatments they are in sense comparable to treatments such as antidepressants or antipsychotics, which are also symptomatic treatments affecting one or other neurotransmitter systems, the difference being that cognitive enhancers are aimed at the 'core' cognitive symptoms of dementia, rather than associated behavioural or psychiatric disturbances.

Cognitive enhancing drugs are thought to act by inhibiting a chemical which breaks down acetylcholine, a neurotransmitter closely involved with memory functions (or, possibly, attentional skills). This chemical is called 'acetylcholinesterase', so these drugs are 'acetylcholinesterase inhibitors' (or 'cholinesterase inhibitors').

The following paragraphs provide some information about the efficacy and side effects of three acetylcholinesterase inhibitors: tacrine (Cognex), donepezil (Aricept) and rivastigmine (Exelon).

Efficacy

Tacrine

There have been a number of published trials of tacrine which have indicated a cognitive performance treatment effect, but this field has been reviewed by the Cochrane Collaboration group (an international organization which surveys medical literature and which is widely seen as producing good quality reviews). Their meta-analysis (a comprehensive review of trials which pools the available data: see also page 44) of the literature found no overall evidence for clear benefit, although there were only a few trials available which allowed pooling of data, and the outcomes of these few trials varied; the group considered that further data was required (Qizilbash *et al.* 1997). In any case, tacrine has a risk of toxic effects on the liver (see section on side effects below) which means it is unlikely to be widely prescribed given the availability of other agents.

Donepezil

Donepezil was approved (for the treatment of mild or moderate dementia in Alzheimer's disease) in the USA in late 1996 and in the EU (including the UK) in the spring of 1997. There are two fundamental trials that have been published. The first of these was essentially a dose ranging study which had relatively small numbers of subjects and, as it turned out, used a low dosage (Rogers *et al.* 1996). Although some measures of cognitive performance indicated a treatment effect, there were others (such as the clinician's rating) which did not show statistically significant differences.

A second and much larger study followed, involving 473 patients who were randomly allocated to receive either placebo, 5mg (milligrams) donepezil, or 10mg donepezil daily for up to 24 weeks; they and all others involved in their care and assessment were blinded as to treatment (Rogers *et al.* 1998). The investigators monitored the patient's progress using various scales, some of which are outlined below. There was no specific scale concerning practical, daily living skills. By and large, the researchers demonstrated modest treatment effects which on most measures reached statistical significance – the one notable failure being a patient-rated measure of quality of life.

One set of figures from the study are given in Table 5.1. These are the response rates derived from the 'Clinician's Interview Based Impression of Change plus care-giver rating'- or CIBIC-Plus (please note that many of the statistical terms and abbreviations used in the following sections are described in Chapter 4).

Before looking at the details of these results, it is worth reflecting on what the practical, real-life implications of such findings may be. This question is raised again at the end of this chapter, but I think it is fair to say that while scales like the CIBIC-Plus attempt to bridge that gap, this kind of data is far from being 'user-friendly'.

Table 5.1 'Improved' Response Rates to Donepezil According to the CIBIC-Plus Scale

	Number in group	% Improved	% Treatment effect	NNT
			(95% CI)	(95% CI)
Placebo	152	11	n/a	n/a
5mg Donepezil	149	26	15 (6.2 – 23.8)	6.7 (16.1 – 4.2)
10mg Donepezil	149	25	14/ (5.5 – 22.5)	7.1/ (18.2 – 4.4)

figures for 5mg and 10mg as follows:

number in treatment group

% response rate

% treatment effect (i.e. net advantage over placebo) with 95% Confidence Interval for treatment effect

Number Need to Treat with 95% CI for NNT.

Source: Rogers, Farlow, Doodyet al. 1998

The figures show that for the patients in this study, who had Alzheimer-type dementia of mild or moderate severity, both 5mg and 10mg of donepezil resulted in an increased response rate (in terms of this clinical rating of impairment – in other words, not an assessment of a person's overall well-being). The advantage over placebo (treatment effect) was roughly 15 per cent: put another way, about one in seven people who were given donepezil were seen as having benefited from it, according to this scale. Note should be made of the confidence intervals, which suggest that the real treatment effect may be much higher – or lower – than the figures suggest.

Results from a test of cognitive abilities (the 70 point ADAS-cog, or Alzheimer's Disease Assessment Scale – cognitive subscale) showed differences as compared to placebo in the *mean* scores of 2.49 points with 5mg, and 2.88 with 10mg. This degree of mean difference is somewhat small, but disguises marked variations in response between individuals. The researchers made a fair attempt to address this problem of using group-based outcome measures such as mean changes by reporting the numbers of people changing by differing degrees according to the assessment scales. Thus, there are reports of the percentage response rates for at least 0 points improvement (i.e. no worsening according to the ADAS-cog); at least a 4 points improvement – which is the minimum expectation of US and European drug approval agencies in respect of this scale; and at least 7 points improvement.

In this trial, 80 per cent of persons given 10mg donepezil did not worsen in terms of the ADAS-cog. However, a very large placebo 'response' (nearly 60 per cent) renders 'non-deterioration' a somewhat unreliable indicator of response in clinical settings, and suggests a net ('real') treatment effect of about 20 per cent. This is broadly the same treatment effect as with 10mg for both the 4 point and 7 point thresholds, suggesting a NNT of around 5. The 5mg dose had a much less marked effect.

Of course, these are somewhat narrow measures of outcome. The patient-rated quality of life scales showed no treatment effect – but such scales are probably too crude a measure to be useful in this area. Clearly, donepezil has some effect in boosting cognitive performance, but this is for a minority of recipients – and there are no indications of which particular persons within the diagnostic group 'mild or moderate dementia in Alzheimer's disease' are going to benefit, and little indication of what the broader, real-life benefits may be. A systematic review (Birks and Melzer 1998) conducted within the Cochrane collaboration drew similar conclusions to those above – that is, donepezil does produce modest improvements but their practical importance is unclear.

Rivastigmine

Rivastigmine received UK approval in the summer of 1998 and shortly afterwards a paper describing one of the main trials was published (Corey-Bloom *et al.* 1998). As with donepezil, this trial involved patients with mild to moderate dementia in Alzheimer's disease. It included a slightly less restricted range of patients than the donepezil trials (which excluded persons with a variety of medical conditions). As with donepezil, a variety of measures were used, again not including a scale to assess daily living skills: no measure of quality of life was attempted.

The data for response rates as measured by the clinical scale (CIBIC-Plus) are not fully presented in the paper, but there appears to a treatment effect of roughly 8 to 9 per cent. Table 5.2 summarizes the data given but it is not entirely clear from the paper whether this relates to all patients who started treatment ('intent-to-treat', see page 49) or to those who stayed in for at least 12 weeks. As explained in Chapter 4, this may mean that some of the figures given would be over-optimistic when compared to those based on intent- to-treat data. Certainly the mean outcome data is not so good for the intent-to-treat subjects. All this would suggest that there are reasons to look very closely at the paper's conclusions (as with donepezil, note the projected range of 'true' treatment effects suggested by the confidence intervals).

Table 5.2 'Improved' Response Rates to Rivastigmine According to the CIBIC-Plus Scale

	Number in group	% Improved	% Treatment effect: 95% CI	NNT: group NNT 95% CI
Placebo	234	16	n/a	n/a
1–4mg	233	25	9% (1.7% – 16.3%)	11.1 (6.1 – 58)
6–12mg	231	24	8% (0.8% – 15.2%)	12.5 (6.6 – 125)

Differences in mean CIBIC-Plus scores were small – the placebo versus 6–12mg group difference just reaching statistical significance. Note that it is not clear as to whether figures are from the larger group of patients who commenced treatment (the figures shown, which achieve significance) or the smaller number of those who completed at least 12 weeks treatment (for which significance is not reached in this analysis). The bottom line is that the paper is not as clear as it might be and that in either case the treatment effect is small.

Data from the ADAS-cog is also provided: looking at the mean difference in scores before and after treatment, the 1–4mg had only a 1.73 point advantage over placebo, whereas the 6–12mg group had a 3.78 point advantage, which was statistically significant.

The paper does not report the percentage response rates according to the ADAS-cog in detail, but states that 'a significantly higher percentage of (rivastigmine) treated patients demonstrated a 4 point or more improvement. A quarter of subjects receiving high-dose treatment (6–12 mg rivastigmine) demonstrated a clinically meaningful improvement (i.e. 4+ points).' (Corey-Bloom et al. 1998, p.58.) Again this data is possibly not 'intent-to-treat' data, so the questions raised above apply here. No placebo response rates are quoted – which means no treatment effect can be estimated – nor is data presented on improvements of 7 points or more.

Results from other measures are also given, being the same or comparable scales as used in the donepezil studies. These appear to follow a similar pattern as for the CIBIC-Plus and ADAS-cog, with mean differences for the higher dose group reaching statistical significance.

Looking at the rivastigmine data overall, it would appear that some statistically significant advantages have been found, but that people receiving rivastigmine may only have about a one in ten chance of a very modest improvement. The paucity of ADAS-cog response rates, especially at the higher 7 point level, perhaps indicates the authors did not have strong data in that area. The issue of which set of patient data is examined (either of all those commencing the trial (intent-to-treat) or of those who remained in the study for at least 12 weeks) complicates interpretation. Furthermore, the reservations made in respect of donepezil regarding translating such outcomes into under-standable, real-life changes apply equally to rivastigmine. Likewise, there appear to be no ways of identifying which patients would be beneficiaries of treatment – something of an issue, given that this may be as few as one in ten.

Side effects

The side effects of tacrine, donepezil and rivastigmine are largely predictable from their action – which is to increase acetylcholine activity. Since acetylcholine plays an important part in the regulation of many organs (such as the stomach and intestines) these drugs have a number of additional effects on bodily functions. The most common effects are nausea, vomiting and diarrhoea. Also predictable from their cholinergic effect is a risk of worsening pre-existing conditions such as heart block, certain respiratory disease such as asthma, oesophagitis or other inflammatory conditions of the oesophagus and stomach. Patients with such conditions were excluded from the donepezil trials, so it is hard to estimate the risks if such persons were treated. The rivastigmine trial was less selective in this respect, although patients with severe or unstable illnesses were excluded.

Tacrine, however, has a further and significant negative effect: it causes abnormalities of liver function. Newer cholinergics such as donepezil and rivastigmine, which differ chemically from tacrine, do not appear to share this difficulty.

Mention should be made of weight loss, which in the case of rivastigmine is reported to be more frequent with higher doses: 21 per cent of those taking 6–12mg, 6 per cent of those on

1–4mg and 2 per cent on placebo lost weight to the extent of at least 7 per cent of their pre-trial weight. This suggests a roughly 18 per cent increased risk of weight loss with higher doses of rivastigmine.

There have also been reports regarding donepezil of psychiatric disturbances such as hallucinations and agitation, which appeared to develop with treatment and remit when treatment was stopped or the dose reduced (Consumers' Association 1998).

Regarding tolerability, both the 5mg donepezil and low dose rivastigmine group (1–4mg) differed little from placebo rates. With 10mg donepezil the discontinuation rate due to adverse events (essentially side effects) was 16 per cent, as compared to 7 per cent for placebo. This is a 9 per cent difference, indicating a 1 in 11 risk of discontinuation with 10mg donepezil due to adverse events. The rivastigmine data is not directly reported in percentage terms, but the comparable figure for the high-dose group (6–12mg) appears to be 28.6 per cent, as compared to 7.2 per cent for placebo. This is a 21.4 per cent difference, indicating a 1 in 4.7 risk of discontinuation with 6–12mg rivastigmine.

TREATMENT WITH COGNITIVE ENHANCERS

Because of the marginal effects of these treatments in many people and the presence of side effects, treatment is not a straightforward matter, as the 'histories' below illustrate.

In this instance it seems that treatment brought mixed blessings – a greater awareness of problems as well as a temporary improvement in some skills. Also to be noted is that the couple were actively seeking treatment and so were keen to press on.

In light of the data about these drugs, it is not a straight-forward matter to predict the value of these drugs for a particular person and whether or not to prescribe them. UK guidance states that treatment with acetylcholinesterase inhibitors should be

Case studies

Jane was an eighty-two-year-old married lady with moderate dementia in Alzheimer's disease. Her family doctor assessed her and wondered if a dementia treatment would be worthwhile, and so after discussing the matter with her and her husband she was referred to a specialist. After a three month trial period – at the start of which Jane experienced some nausea – it appeared that although there had been an initial improvement in some skills this had not been sustained and that overall there had been no real benefit. Although both she and her husband were disappointed with this, they both accepted that her treatment should be discontinued.

Richard was a sixty-nine-year-old retired business man with mild to moderate dementia in Alzheimer's disease. When his wife noticed media reports about dementia treatments they both discussed the possibility of a trial of treatment with their family doctor and this led to medication being given. After several months Richard and his wife reported an increased ability to concentrate with some improvement in memory and overall abilities. Whilst this was beneficial in a number of ways, Richard became more aware of some financial difficulties and at times became distressed about this. On the other hand, he experienced no physical side effects and overall Richard and his wife were pleased with the outcome, which was of modest improvement in several areas of mental functioning. After a further six months, some slight deterioration was apparent, but it was agreed to continue with treatment for the time being.

initiated and supervised by a specialist (such as a psychiatrist for older adults). It is also clear that a full assessment of the patient's suitability should be made before treatment is considered. This will include making some cognitive assessments to act as a baseline – for example, the widely used Mini-Mental State (Folstein *et al.* 1975). This will help clinicians in judging whether or not a person's cognitive impairment falls within the mild to moderate range of the clinical trials (a Mini-Mental State score of 10–26 would suggest this).

Yet above and beyond any formal criteria, it is vital that an appraisal is made about the potential overall impact of a trial of treatment upon the individual. If treatment is considered a possibility, it will also be important to ensure that the patient (so far as is possible) and his or her carers understand that this would be a trial of treatment, which would be discontinued if of no benefit.

For both donepezil and rivastigmine it would seem best to aim for the highest tolerable dose: but to reach this gradually (e.g. spacing dose increases by at least two weeks) so as to minimize side effects. The patient should then be formally re-assessed – after twelve weeks or so – to see if any gains have been made in comparison to their baseline status. If they have, and it is agreed that overall the person has benefited, then treatment should probably continue until it does not appear to be appropriate or becomes unsafe.

If treatment does not seem to have helped it should be stopped – although if a sudden deterioration then occurs it may be justifiable to repeat the trial of treatment, as the patient may be a responder after all. Naturally such a decision will not be easy, especially when the differences between response and non-response are small, and given that (despite some accounts) people with dementia in Alzheimer's disease do not steadily and invariably decline.

COGNITIVE ENHANCERS – ARE THEY WORTH IT?

Concerning tacrine, there would seem to be little merit in prescribing it (where available) as a first line agent, given the conclusions of the Cochrane review of its unclear value and the significant safety concerns. Whether it could be justified as a second line therapy after failure with donepezil or rivastigmine is also questionable: as yet, we have no evidence about the chances of a person who has not been helped by one of these agents then responding to another cholinesterase inhibitor.

Regarding the currently narrow evidence base for donepezil, the general consensus by reviewers of the first, smaller study was that it did not clearly demonstrate a treatment benefit. By contrast, although there have been fewer reviews (to date) of the 1998 paper, there seems to be an acceptance that the treatment effect as measured by some scales has reached statistical significance. There are some reported concerns regarding psychiatric side effects, although the risk of these has not been quantified and it should be acknowledged that widely prescribed drugs such as antidepressants or antipsychotics can cause psychotic or confusional problems.

Turning to rivastigmine, it is tempting to make some comparisons with donepezil (not least because the authors of the rivastigmine paper do so). However, great caution should be taken in such comparisons, as there may be crucial differences in the populations studied; indeed, the rivastigmine subjects did include those with a wider range of medical disorders and were slightly older, which may be at least part of the explanation for the apparently lower tolerability and lower response rates with rivastigmine as reported from this one trial. It is also difficult to draw comparisons between the two treatments because of the differences in data presentation.

Overall, there does seem to be evidence of some measurable improvement associated with acetylcholinesterase inhibitor treatments. What is less obvious is the real significance of such changes. The comments regarding the lack of specific estimates of practical daily living skills apply to both donepezil and rivastigmine: this is an unfortunate gap.

Clinical trials tend to measure clinical outcome with scales which are deliberately analytic; that is, for reasons of good science, they aim for precise (i.e. narrow) answers. By contrast, it is much harder to assess overall benefit to the person, by which I mean the balance of good and adverse effects of a treatment. To be fair, some of the studies have made some attempts at this, and it is debatable how well holistic assessments can result in data susceptible to the usual statistics (e.g. summation, averaging or treatment effects). The lack of useful data on quality of life is therefore a real problem (if not an uncommon one) for although this is clearly a difficult 'thing' to measure, it is at the same time very important. After all, it is the *person* with dementia who receives such treatment, and he or she remains a whole person throughout the course of their illness, whatever difficulties others may have in communicating with them.

There is no clinical evidence that cholinesterase inhibitors in any way *cure* dementia, or even arrest decline: they appear to be able to 'buy' a temporary reversal or halting of decline for a proportion of persons who receive them. (There has been speculation that these agents may affect the underlying pathology – specifically, the deposition of abnormal amyloid protein. Such suggestions will require much more evidence before gaining general acceptance.) It is also thought that cholinesterase inhibitors may treat other dementia-related problems, such as behavioural disturbance, possibly even having an antipsychotic effect; again, clinical trial evidence for this is lacking (and such claims need to be set against the reports of treatment-induced disturbance).

The issue of treatment costs with these agents is real – and seems unlikely to diminish if and when further drugs are launched onto the markets. It is interesting to note that some other nations, such as Australia, require drug companies to submit cost-benefit analyses as part of submissions for new drug approvals. In many ways this is to be welcomed, so long as the result is not to deprive patients of treatments in new areas – such as the dementias, through 'shifting the goal posts' for such treatments. Quite clearly, though, the issue of the costs of new drugs for new indications has implications for health care expenditure (not just due to drug but also diagnosis and monitoring costs); governments may not be able to allow the current systems to continue as they now stand.

From a personal viewpoint – and value judgements are involved here – for hitherto untreatable aspects of a condition which causes so much disability and distress, even a 1 in 10 chance of modest gains such as these would be of some value, as long as concerns that the person as a whole should be considered in assessing outcome or of the possibility of side effects are borne in mind. Such an opinion is not been shared by everyone, and I am aware of the possible message of the confidence intervals on the outcome data, which is that it is not beyond the bounds of possibility that these treatments have scarcely any effect at all. The reviewers in the UK Drugs and Therapeutics Bulletin article which was quoted earlier 'remained unconvinced of the value of donepezil' (Consumers Association 1998); there has been no review yet of rivastigmine. Finally, the negative conclusions of the meta-analysis of tacrine must add to the caution over this group of agents, despite the difficulties in finding suitable trials and the possibility that the newer treatments may be more effective.

POSSIBLE TREATMENTS FOR DEMENTIA PATHOLOGIES

The cognitive enhancing drugs described in the previous section might be able to provide modest symptomatic improvement in some aspects of dementia; they do not treat the underlying pathologies. But there are other drugs which may do so: they are a highly diverse group of medications, some of which have been available for many years, but not necessarily used in dementia; others are new products. There is not much good quality evidence about many of these treatments, but some of these drugs may have some benefit. On the whole, these possible gains are in terms of slowing the rate of decline rather than improving the person's current status. This would seem to suggest such treatments should be commenced sooner rather than later.

Individual treatments: Efficacy and side effects

Aspirin

Aspirin is very familiar medication (of herbal ancestry, namely extract of willow bark). At doses used for pain relief, it also has anti-inflammatory properties and, at lower doses, is able to reduce the 'stickiness' of certain blood cells (platelets) which are involved in the formation of blood clots. This latter effect is thought to underlie aspirin's proven value in reducing the risk of repeat heart attacks and strokes where infarction has occurred. Given the association between stroke disease and vascular dementia, there may be grounds to think low dose aspirin could be of value. There is also the possibility of an effect in other dementias, such as Alzheimer's, where there is evidence for a circulatory component to the pathology. Concerning the anti-inflammatory properties of aspirin, and of other drugs, such as ibuprofen (called Non-Steroidal Anti-Inflammatory Drugs, or NSAIDs), there is a possibility that by slowing inflammatory reactions the extent of brain tissue damage in dementia may be reduced (Breitner *et al.* 1994).

Aspirin has not been extensively studied in dementia, but two studies, which were community surveys rather than controlled trials, came to differing conclusions as to whether it confers a modest benefit or not (Henderson *et al.* 1997; Stürmer *et al.* 1996). Aspirin does carry risks of irritation of the lining of the gut – for example, in the stomach – and this can lead to blood loss. This is more of a problem with higher dose aspirin, and as yet there is no evidence to warrant routine prescription of higher dose aspirin. Regarding low dose aspirin, it is of course no coincidence that many people diagnosed with vascular dementia are receiving aspirin already for other circulatory problems. There is no evidence to date which supports routine use of aspirin in Alzheimer's disease.

Extract of Ginkgo biloba

Another treatment, this time more obviously herbal in origin, is Extract of Ginkgo biloba (EGb). This has been prescribed for some time (especially in continental Europe) for a variety of neurological problems including dementia. Its mechanisms of action are not entirely clear, but may be around reducing free radical activity, thereby slowing the rate of damage to neurones through excessive oxidation (free radicals are body chemicals implicated in a variety of conditions; tissue damage occurs when their activity is not sufficiently controlled). A review published in 1992 compared EGb to hydergine (see below) and found comparable efficacy but noted various problems with the published evidence as it then stood (Kleijnen and Knipschild 1992).

A more recent placebo controlled trial found that on some measures, whereas patients treated with placebo deteriorated over the 12 months study period, patients taking 120mg daily of EGb (as three doses of 40mg) did not deteriorate, according to the measures used (Le Bars *et al.* 1997). The Numbers Needed to Treat to achieve an advantage over placebo of 4 points on the ADAS-cog (see page 54) was about 8 for all patients, falling to 5.3 for Alzheimer patients. These findings were not universal: a clinician scale (the CIBIC-plus; see page 53) did not detect any difference. However, a carer scale did show benefit. The study did not use a quality of life scale. Nonetheless, given that EGb has few known adverse side effects, this study would appear to indicate this medication has useful potential in both Alzheimer and vascular dementia.

Vitamin E

Vitamin E (or alpha-tocopherol), another anti-oxidant or free radical inhibitor has been suggested as a dementia treatment. A recent trial seemed to show some benefit to persons with Alzheimer type dementia, in terms of reduced risk of moving to an institution (Sano *et al.* 1997). A reviewer noted some difficulties with this conclusion, as a significant difference only emerged after adjustments were made to take account of differences between the treatment groups (Hirsch 1997). There is also the issue of whether supplementary vitamin treatment has any role if an adequate diet is taken. However, the study did use a clear cut and practical outcome measure – whereas the more sophisticated measures of cognitive function (such as those quoted for EGb and donepezil) cannot so easily be translated into clinical practice. Although the case for routine use of vitamin E in Alzheimer's remains unproven it does not appear to have adverse effects at the dose used in this study (1000IU twice daily).

Selegiline

The vitamin E study quoted above also examined the effects of selegiline, an agent which has been used in Parkinson's disease with the aim of slowing progression in that condition: selegiline is thought to have anti-oxidant properties. The study did suggest a small benefit, but with similar uncertainties as with vitamin E. Selegiline does have interactions with various medications, including certain antidepressants (e.g. moclobemide and various SSRIs). Until a fuller picture of its benefits and risks is obtained, it would not seem appropriate for use in dementia.

Hydergine

One treatment which has been available for many years but has fallen somewhat into abeyance, at least in the UK, is Hydergine. This drug, or rather combination of compounds called co-dergocrine mesylate, is related to the naturally derived substance ergot. It has actions on several neurotransmitters, but may also have therapeutic effect through improving cerebral metabolism (Wadworth and Crisp 1992). There is some debate over whether this drug is truly neuroprotective (i.e. slows the rate of damage to neurones), or should be considered as a candidate cognitive enhancer. A review of treatment trials found indications of a real but very small advantage over placebo, with speculation that doses higher than the current approved maximum (4.5 mg daily in the UK) may be more effective (Schneider and Olin 1994). Within the 4.5mg limit, side effects are said to be infrequent, but include abdominal discomfort and flushing. The overall place of hydergine in dementia treatment is still unclear – perhaps the advent of new and expensive treatments will promote its reappraisal.

Calcium channel blocking drugs

The suggestion that excessive flow of calcium ions into neurones may be toxic has prompted studies of calcium channel blocking drugs – which are normally used to treat heart conditions. Unfortunately, the current Cochrane Collaboration review of one such agent – nimodipine – found no clear evidence for benefit in dementia (Qizilbash, Arrieta and Birks 1997). It should be added that the reviewers seemed to have encountered difficulties similar to those with tacrine – namely, a lack of studies with data suitable for pooling, and noted that further studies may alter the current balance of evidence. At any rate, there is no current basis for the use in dementia of calcium channel blocking agents such as nimodipine outside of clinical trials.

Drugs currently being developed

There are other anti-dementia drugs under development which have yet to be approved and marketed: these include propentophylline, a drug which, like Extract of Ginkgo biloba, may have anti-oxidant properties and may have other neuro-protective effects. There have been a number of published trials, including a twelve month placebo controlled trial (Marcusson *et al.* 1997). The study involved patients with dementia of any sub-type, but of only mild to moderate severity. Looking at the results for all dementia patients, statistically significant differences were found on most measures. The difference was small – about a five per cent advantage according to one of the cognitive scales. Carer ratings also showed a modest advantage with propentophylline. Nausea, dizziness, abdominal pain and headache were all about five per cent more common with propentophylline than placebo. As with all such new medications, the numbers of persons studied makes predictions regarding rarer adverse events somewhat difficult.

Overall, propentophylline may be of value, but many of the scales used are different from those in other studies, and the data as presented does not allow response rates to be readily calculated, thus making comparisons with other treatments difficult. There is no data on the long-term effects of propentophylline – especially as to whether it has any sustained effect in slowing decline. These questions may be addressed, assuming the drug does become available.

There is speculation that oestrogens – as found in hormone replacement therapy – may reduce the severity of dementia. Oestrogens may have a role in promoting tissue repair and so reduce the effects of damaging pathological processes, but there is no indication as yet to establish these hormones as having a certain place in dementia therapy.

CONCLUSIONS: CAN DRUGS STOP DEMENTIA?

There are some recurrent themes which emerge from this quick tour of a selection of the various potential treatments for persons with dementia. A number of these compounds are thought to act by reducing the damage caused by excessive free radical activity or oxidation. The presence of herbal treatments, or of drugs in some way related to natural biological substances is also interesting. Just how specific the actions of these agents may be to dementia pathology, as opposed to having general effects which include a possible slowing of dementia is as yet unclear. Again, knowledge of how such drugs may impact upon individual persons and their well-being is by and large absent. It is perhaps the provisional and evolving state of evidence about these compounds which is so striking – even for such well known drugs as aspirin.

Where there is evidence for efficacy, this is typically of a very modest degree. This should not be taken to mean that such an effect is not significant. If a drug – one of these, or another – does emerge as having a neuroprotective function, then over the time period of most trials such effects are bound to be small. Even if a drug entirely arrested the dementia process, unless the drug had some cognitive enhancing effect it could never have more impact than reversing the equivalent amount of normal decline over the duration of the study. Furthermore, there is usually a significant placebo response in dementia trials (as in most other treatment trials), which may then diminish the calculated effect size when comparing the active drug to placebo.

Of the treatments currently available, there does appear to be evidence to support the use of Extract of Ginkgo biloba in persons with dementia (in the UK this preparation is not a 'prescription only medicine' and is available through various health retail outlets). Low dose aspirin might be considered for persons with vascular dementia – persons with a history of stroke (where infarction has occurred) or heart attack (myocardial infarction) are potential candidates for aspirin in any case. Hydergine may be of value, but the extent and nature of any benefit will need to be compared with the benefits of other treatments. Vitamin E appears to be reasonably safe, but there is not convincing evidence of its therapeutic value.

Turning to how the benefits of such drugs might be assessed, whereas with cognitive enhancing agents it is possible to monitor for improvement in individual patients, assessing the outcome in this group of drugs is somewhat difficult, as 'reduced decline' is the hoped-for outcome. Since it is hard to give specific prognoses for individual patients it will be difficult to know if the long-term outcome has been better than it would have been without treatment. Indeed, this type of treatment is essentially preventative (of deterioration, not the disease itself) and usually such treatments are given on the grounds of large prospective trial data, on the basis that treating many persons falling into an 'at-risk' group will benefit some by reducing further illness. This is the philosophy behind policies such as the prescription of low dose aspirin to all those who have had a heart attack, in the hope of reducing the risk of further heart attacks.

It may be that in a few years persons with many forms of dementia will routinely receive such prophylactic medication (perhaps even aspirin itself). This would have implications for clinicians, in terms of early diagnosis and intervention – and depending on the balance of evidence, could mean the widespread prescription of proven – but sometimes costly – medications.

Chapter 6

Antipsychotics and Dementia

BACKGROUND

Of all the different kinds of drugs given to persons with dementia, antipsychotics have been the most controversial. Concerns over their excessive use in nursing homes – raised vociferously in the US – led to legislative measures which now determine the manner of their use in that country. The US legislation (OBRA-87) has been dealt with in more detail in the introduction.

The principles of drug treatment outlined in Chapter 3 provide some useful background to this topic: I want to re-emphasize here the need to maintain a broad perspective to care, which is focused on the person as a whole in their care environment, rather than just 'problem behaviours' or 'symptoms'. Thus, treatment with drugs such as antipsychotics may occasionally be of value, but is only one element of caring for a person affected by dementia.

Antipsychotic treatment has been prescribed to persons with dementia since the 1950s, when such drugs first became available. They continue to be prescribed, with proportions of up to one half of nursing home residents receiving such medications, with lower levels in residential homes (reported as 23% in some London homes in 1986) and lower still in community settings (Mann, Graham and Ashby 1986).

The likelihood of receiving such medication in a nursing home may have more to do with the size of the home or prescriber's characteristic than the presence or absence of a dementia syndrome. Furthermore, a 1986 survey of residential homes found substantial numbers of persons with unrecognized depressive symptoms (Mann, Graham and Ashby 1986; Ray, Federspiel and Schaffner 1980).

Antipsychotics are a large group of drugs grouped together by conventions of clinical use, rather than structural similarities (there are other terms for this group of drugs, including 'neuroleptics' and 'major tranquillizers'. There used to be a simple model of how such drugs worked – namely, by blocking dopamine receptors, but this link has been disproven by the evidence that 'novel' antipsychotics such as clozapine or quetiapine are antipsychotic drugs with a serotonin blocking action which seems to operate alongside a more selective dopamine blocking activity. This means that novel anti-psychotics carry a lower risk of causing side effects such as parkinsonism (see page 80) – though evidence for this in persons affected by dementia is not available.

The antipsychotic effects of these drugs – which are reductions in delusions or hallucinations – do not come about immediately, but after a week or so. Thus, prescribing clinicians should not expect to see an immediate antipsychotic effect – they should wait for at least a week before judging a particular dosage or drug ineffective. These drugs do have other effects – which are defined as side effects if they are unwanted, but may at times be seen as beneficial. For example sedation – due to blockade of receptors for a neurotransmitter called histamine – may be considered of value if there is marked agitation or sleep difficulties.

I will briefly mention long-acting injections (called 'depot injections') which are available for a small number of antipsychotics. These consist of the active drug in combination with a long fatty acid chain, suspended in an oily base: the idea is that the active drug is slowly released from the site of the injection over a period of several weeks. The fact that such preparations may have long-lasting effects would suggest considerable caution in their use in persons with dementia, especially those who are frail. So although depot injections are successfully used in treating other conditions such as schizophrenia, their role in dementia treatment is probably very limited.

EFFICACY

Case study

Daniel was a seventy-five-year old man diagnosed with severe mixed dementia (vascular and Alzheimer's disease). He had a history of aggressiveness towards his wife over the last year, but in the last two months this had become much more frequent. He was also up and restless most nights. His wife, exhausted and frightened, was felt to be at definite risk. He was compulsorily admitted to hospital under mental health legislation. For the first few days he was not aggressive, although very disoriented and forgetful. He then started to show hostility and this escalated into physical violence, despite staff interventions. He was prescribed 0.5mg haloperidol which seemed to help, in that he became less aggressive. This was given on a regular basis (twice daily), but after a few days he began to show signs of stiffness and excessive salivation. The dose was reduced to once daily, and the stiffness resolved. He went on leave with additional support at home, and his wife joined a carer support group. Eventually he was discharged and went home.

Case study continued

However, about two months after commencing haloperidol, the psychiatrist reviewing him noticed abnormal movements of his face, which were considered to be side effects (tardive dyskinesia). The haloperidol was stopped: the abnormal movements briefly became worse, but then largely disappeared. Verbal aggression returned to some extent, but his wife had developed ways to identify irritants and to defuse most situations, without herself becoming tense and angry – a problem which she now acknowledged. Overall, although the situation was still stressful and not risk free, it was sustainable.

Although such severe aggression is not typical, it is far from rare, and tranquillizing medication of some kind often appears to be unavoidable – especially if it is hoped that the person with dementia will be able to return home in the end. In this instance an eventual alternative to medication was found. This will not always be possible, but the continued prescribing of such drugs needs to be kept under continual review.

How successful are antipsychotics in treating dementia-related problems? The evidence available is not extensive, and much of it is in the form of open trials; even several of the double blind placebo controlled trials have significant methodology problems. There is also the question of the definition of the terms used in the trials – for example agitation, including aggression, has been defined and assessed with varying precision. Antipsychotics are also given to treat psychotic symptoms such as hallucinations or delusions. It is important to be sure that the target problem (e.g. hallucinations) is sufficiently serious to merit intervention: indeed, hallucinations and delusions experienced by persons with dementia – such as seeing deceased relatives or believing one is at home – may be comforting rather than distressing.

Various reviews of this field have been undertaken (including a meta-analysis: Schneider, Pollock and Lyness 1990) of clinical trials studying the impact of antipsychotics on 'agitation' in dementia (Borson and Rishkind 1997; Lantz and Marin 1996;Tariot 1996). In Schneider's paper, all relevant trials conducted before 1990 were examined and the results from those fulfilling certain quality criteria – six in all from 1962 to 1982 – were pooled. The conclusion was that the net benefit of low dose antipsychotics over placebo was 18 per cent – for every 100 patients given antipsychotics, 18 would have become less agitated as a result (or a NNT of 5.5, see page 46).

Most reviewers since 1990 have agreed with the broad conclusions of this meta-analysis, namely that antipsychotics in dementia are of modest clinical value This apparent gain is generally in terms of observed behaviour or decreased agitation – and does not reflect the person's overall well-being or quality of life. Schneider *et al.* and other authors (Devanand and Levy 1995) have observed that the studies quoted did not take into account clinical worsening or any side effects – making the overall impact on the individual hard to assess. The studies also included a mix of dementia sub-types and did not take account of patients who dropped out of the trial before completion. In other words, the studies did not use current best practice in research – not surprisingly, since the most recent study was published in 1982, which is indicative of the lack of research available.

An earlier review had come to much the same conclusion and suggested that suspiciousness, hallucinations, sleeplessness and agitated behaviours such as excitement, hostility, belligerence or emotional instability were the most likely to be reduced by antipsychotics (Risse and Barnes 1986). In contrast, repetitive behaviours such as pacing or calling out appeared to be less responsive to treatment. It should be noted, however, that a systematic review of the efficacy of thioridazine, a widely used antipsychotic, was unable to identify sufficient evidence to justify its use in people with dementia (Kirchner, Kelly and Harvey 1998).

There have been a number of studies comparing different antipsychotics, the overall conclusion of reviewers being that no particular drug appears to be superior to another. Schneider *et al.* (1990) also report a substantial placebo effect – of the order of 40 – 50 per cent. This suggests that 'non-specific interventions are effective' for many patients. Together with the treatment effect, this suggests that for about 70 per cent of people with dementia given antipsychotics in a clinical setting, problems such as agitation or aggression would diminish – but that this would be due to the drug itself in only a proportion (roughly one third) of 'responders'. To put it another way, 'much of the time, neuroleptics do not control agitation' (Schneider, Pollock and Lyness 1991). These figures may well explain how anti-psychotics seem at first to make a difference in dementia, yet their performance is nothing like so impressive in the longer term, and when compared to placebo. Furthermore, all this is based upon a few narrow measures of symptoms or behaviours which tell us little or nothing about the overall impact of such drugs.

The various reviewers nonetheless affirm the benefits of the use of antipsychotics: and they urge caution in turning to other medications whose efficacy and side effects have yet to be adequately researched. The high placebo response rate and low treatment effect mean that real differences between drugs given for agitation in dementia may be hard to detect. They conclude that the results of any treatment trial which does not include a placebo group should be viewed with caution.

A further aspect of a high placebo response rate could be that, since treatment will seem to be effective, there will be a strong temptation to continue it, even though there will be a significant number of persons remaining on a drug which in reality is useless to them. It is possible that after a period of time even 'true' responders may no longer require medication – as suggested by the 1966 study mentioned in Chapter 1 (Barton and Hurst 1966).

The broad conclusions of the Barton paper appear to have been confirmed by a study in nursing home settings of patients suffering from dementia who had been taking antipsychotics (Bridges-Parlet *et al.* 1997). In this study, some of the residents had their antipsychotics withdrawn under blinded and controlled conditions (i.e. all patients were given medication identical in appearance, but some of these were given placebo whilst others continued to take antipsychotics). Of the 22 patients who were withdrawn, only 2 exhibited problem behaviours requiring removal from the study, and half of these patients were able to remain off antipsychotic medication for a mean minimum period of forty weeks. Moreover, most patients who showed physically aggressive behaviour before the withdrawal trial began, showed little change in behaviour throughout the duration of the trial. Another (uncontrolled) study also reported few adverse results from withdrawal – indeed, it found improvement in terms of mood ratings (Thapa *et al.* 1994).

I should add that these studies had limitations: perhaps most importantly – as the authors themselves point out – the subjects were not randomly selected. This could mean that patients who were included tended to be those on lower doses of medication or for whom there was less staff concern about the risks of withdrawing treatment. The 1997 study (Bridges-Parlet *et al.*), although well designed, is identified as a pilot study, and indeed the number of participants is small for what is a kind of treatment trial in reverse (calculations by Schneider *et al.* (1990) of the sample size needed to avoid falsely concluding there was no treatment effect (a 'Type II' error; see page 45) suggested around 190 subjects would be required). The 1994 study by Thapa *et al.* also had other drawbacks, apart from the lack of a control group or blinding, namely the lack of detail as to the range of mental health problems the study population were suffering from – in particular, the proportion who could be diagnosed as suffering from dementia.

Despite the limitations of these withdrawal studies, they, in combination with data from placebo controlled treatment trials, strongly suggest that while antipsychotics are of value to some patients, they offer little to most patients, and that substantial numbers of persons with dementia may be receiving anti-psychotics on a continuing basis without benefit. As has already been noted, these recent studies have been foreshadowed by research conducted more than thirty years ago (see page 8), so such conclusions should not come as any surprise.

SIDE EFFECTS

As mentioned above, antipsychotics could nowadays be divided into two broad categories: 'conventional' and 'novel' according to whether or not they have side effects linked to the blocking actions of antipsychotics on dopamine activity in certain parts of the brain. One such side effect is parkinsonism (so called because of a resemblance to Parkinson's disease): it includes mental symptoms such as slowed thought, depression and worsening of cognitive impairment, as well as physical signs such as rigid muscle tone, tremor, shuffling gait, reduced facial expression and excessive salivation. But such effects on dopamine are by no means the end of the story. Many antipsychotics – including some novel ones – have blocking actions on other neuro-transmitters' receptors, leading to a range of problems for their recipients.

Side effects such as parkinsonism are linked to processes within the nervous system which regulate voluntary movement. The drugs affect what is called the 'extra- pyramidal system' (there are structures running through the spinal cord called the 'pyramids' on account of their appearance on cross-section: they contain nerve fibres conveying signals for voluntary acts from the brain to the muscles). The extrapyramidal system refers, as the name implies, to structures *outside* the pyramidal system but which influence the signals passing through it. Blocking the actions of dopamine in this 'extra-pyramidal' system causes side effects such as disorders of muscle tone and movement which are termed extrapyramidal side effects – EPSE for short.

It is clear that dopamine has a key role in causing EPSE; but acetylcholine, too, is a significant transmitter involved with this system, and appears to have a counter balancing effect to dopamine. Thus, the parkinsonian effects of dopamine blockade can be reduced by blocking acetylcholine with anticholinergic drugs such as procyclidine (imagine a pair of scales – if you add weight on one side you will need to add a weight to the other in order to keep a balance).

Some antipsychotics have a marked anticholinergic effect, and so are less prone to cause EPSEs. Conventional antipsychotics with relatively focused dopamine-blocking action are sometimes termed 'high potency'; those with marked effects on a variety of receptors are termed 'low potency'. There is some evidence that the counterbalancing relationship between acetylcholine and dopamine extends beyond the extrapyramidal system: for example, drugs promoting dopamine activity, such as antiparkinsonian agents, can have psychotic side effects. Conversely, the possibility that psychotic symptoms might be reduced by promoting acetylcholine function is currently being explored (Borson and Rishkind 1997; Cummings and Kaufer 1996).

There are a number of other extrapyramidal side effects, apart from the parkinsonian syndrome. These include: acute muscle spasms (or 'dystonias', particularly of the neck, back or eye muscles); and an unsettling sensation of restlessness, often causing the person to become restless (called akathisia, derived from the Greek for chair – as in 'I can't sit down'). Akathisia is described as including anxiety and jitteriness – and may be linked to increased disturbance and aggression. Such disturbances might lead carers and clinicians to give higher doses of medication – when the medication is actually making matters worse, not better. These side effects may emerge quite soon after commencing treatment, even after a few days (Sweet *et al.* 1994).

There is one further type of extra-pyramidal side effect to describe, and that is involuntary movements (or 'dyskinesia') affecting the mouth and face, the trunk, or legs – even the respiratory muscles including the diaphragm. These dyskinesias usually develop later on in treatment, that is, they are 'tardive'. They appear to be caused by imbalances between different sub-types of dopamine receptors, and in part it seems there is a 'rebound' overcompensation for the dopamine blocking effect.

Tardive dyskinesia has the unfortunate tendency to become worse after drug withdrawal or dose reduction. Tardive dyskinesia is also made worse by anticholinergic drugs, which reduce parkinsonian side effects (this fits the model of acetylcholine being in counterbalance to dopamine). There is also concern that concurrent use of anticholinergic drugs and antipsychotics may increase the risk of tardive dyskinesia (TD). In the long term, TD usually subsides after withdrawing the offending drug – but not always. In other words, this is a 'side effect' which may persist for years after the causative drug has been withdrawn – indeed, most elderly persons suffering from TD continue to have symptoms after five years (Wood and Castleton 1991). There is evidence that increasing age and female sex are risk factors for tardive dyskinesia – something of a problem, given the typical profile of people affected by dementia. Other risk factors for TD may include early development of parkinsonian symptoms, previous treatment with antipsychotics, history of alcohol abuse, pre-existing movement disorder and doses of more than 3mg of haloperidol or 150mg chlorpromazine equivalents (Lantz and Marin 1996; Pollock and Mulsant 1995). It is not hard to see that needlessly prolonged treatment could carry serious implications for patients receiving antipsychotic medications.

There would be less cause for concern if these extra-pyramidal side effects were rare. Unfortunately, they are all too common. Parkinsonism alone may occur in up to 75 per cent of patients and may persist for up to 36 weeks after drug discontinuation. Estimates for the risk of tardive dyskinesias vary within a range of roughly one-quarter to nearly one half, even with fairly low doses (Pollock and Mulsant 1995).

Antipsychotics have other side effects as well; these are summarized in Appendix I. There is some evidence of an association between antipsychotics and more rapid cognitive decline, but this has not been confirmed (McShane *et al.* 1997). One study reported a two-fold increase in the risk of fractured femur amongst nursing home residents given antipsychotics – but similar risks were linked to long-acting sedatives or anti-anxiety drugs and to tricyclic antidepressants (Ray *et al.* 1987). It should also be realised that antipsychotics do not produce all these side effects in all patients. On the whole, drugs from within the same chemical class have similar side effect profiles; Appendix II provides some information about specific antipsychotics.

Concerning drug interactions, clinicians should consult sources of up-to-date prescribing information such as product data sheets, or the British National Formulary. Appendix III provides such information in summary.

The increased confusion that John experienced could have been linked to his drug treatment in various ways: for example, drugs such as chlorpromazine and especially procyclidine can cause this directly through their anticholinergic effects. Other possibilities are compromising blood circulation to the brain (adrenergic blockade causing hypotension) or constipation (anticholinergic effects once more).

Case study

John was an eighty-four-year-old widower with severe dementia in Alzheimer's disease. He had been cared for at a residential home for many years and his dementia had worsened over time. He was still able to feed himself, but required assistance with washing and dressing. He was physically aggressive to female staff giving such care, and could also hit out at female residents and staff at other times, especially later in the day. He had been on a low dose of thioridazine when he came to the home and this was increased. His aggression diminished, but then returned. He was given chlorpromazine instead but became unsteady, though still aggressive and if anything more restless. He developed stiffness and shaking, side effects of chlorpromazine, and these were treated with procyclidine. His confusion worsened and hospital admission was arranged. Physical examination revealed he had low blood pressure and constipation, both of which resolved after discontinuing medication. His confusion and wandering also reduced and again were in part due to other side effects of the medication. Eventually, he was successfully cared for in a specialist setting with some male staff and with only occasional medication.

ARE ANTIPSYCHOTICS AND DEMENTIA A CAUSE FOR CONCERN?

Conventional antipsychotics are undoubtedly used as a mainstay of drug treatment for many dementia patients – hopefully after and alongside non-drug interventions. Yet there must remain some concern that they are too often used as an automatic response and as the principle intervention. Such an approach must be considered questionable, given the evidence (much of it quite old) about these drugs when prescribed to persons with dementia. There is evidence for some efficacy – but only in about one fifth of recipients and not in all the problems for which such treatment may be given. There is also evidence to suggest that long-term treatment for dementia-related problems is not usually required. There are real grounds for concern when it comes to side effects, particularly when the widely prescribed conventional antipsychotics are given to persons with dementia. Faced with only a one in five chance of a real response and yet a 50 per cent chance of inducing unpleasant mental and physical side effects, clinicians may well pause before initiating such treatments. As described elsewhere in this guide, the fact that these drugs were the early and prime focus of specific US legislation (OBRA-87) is testimony to the fine balance between the pros and cons of such treatments. It is questionable how much support there would be for the widespread use of drugs such as chlorpromazine and thioridazine if they were being launched now (see Kirchner, Kelly and Harvey 1998).

By contrast, the novel antipsychotics do not appear to carry risks associated with parkinsonian symptoms – but several do have other significant side effects. In time, evidence may become available for their efficacy and safety in dementia but pending this, clinicians would be wise to bear in mind the lack of evidence to date and only to use them with the same caution as other antipsychotics.

It is therefore not surprising that clinicians have tried alternatives to antipsychotics in treating emotional, behavioural or other psychiatric problems in persons with dementia, and it is to such treatments that I turn in the following chapter.

Chapter 7

Other Drug Treatments For Dementia

This chapter describes various other drugs which can be pre-scribed for emotional or behavioural problems in dementia, which include antidepressants, anti-anxiety agents and mood stabilizers.

ANTIDEPRESSANTS: BACKGROUND

It is well recognized that dementia is often associated with depressive syndromes. Mood disorders are more common amongst persons with dementia and there is some evidence of deficiencies in the neurotransmitters linked to depression. It would also be reasonable to suppose that people with dementia may become distressed at their situation, especially in the earliest and more insightful stages of dementia, and also that persons with a history of mood disorder may have further problems after a dementia syndrome becomes apparent.

Estimates of the occurrence of major depression in people with dementia range from 5 to 15 per cent, whilst depressive symptoms may occur at some time in up to 50 per cent of persons with dementia. 'Minor depression' may be present in 25 per cent of persons with dementia. The distinction between depressive symptoms and a depressive *disorder* (especially major depression) may be important when it comes to treatment: a depressive disorder is a set of problems which includes more or less continuously low mood for at least several weeks (and usually months); depressive symptoms include brief periods of unhappiness or apathy. Likewise, people affected by dementia may have depressive problems for a period of time, but rarely in the long term. People with dementia (especially of a vascular type) may be prone to sudden changes in mood ('lability of mood') which may include tearfulness or agitation. One could speculate as to why this is so: brain pathology may well play a part (this problem is often prominent in people who have suffered strokes) but other possibilities could well include the person's reactions to their own condition and their interactions with others.

There is evidence that, along with other psychiatric symptoms, depression appears to be commoner amongst persons with dementia who live in residential settings (Mann, Graham and Ashby 1986). It is not clear whether this is due to greater numbers of people with such problems requiring care, or if residential care was in some way a causative factor in their depression.

Depression can manifest as a dementia syndrome, yet the cognitive and functional problems taken for dementia resolve upon treatment for depression – this phenomenon has earned the sobriquet 'pseudo-dementia'. It seems now, however, that the true picture is not this simple. People successfully treated for 'pseudo-dementia' are at a higher risk of developing true dementia later – and the original cognitive problems do not always fully resolve. Another clue comes from people who develop depression for the first time in later life, and tend to have pathological changes similar to those in dementia, but to a lesser degree. Overall, it would seem that attempting to base treatment upon a strict dichotomy between depression and dementia is unlikely to be helpful.

There are also associations between other brain disorders and disturbances of mood. Persons with frontal lobe dementia often have symptoms suggestive of depression, such as apathy and inactivity. Parkinson's disease is associated with psychological problems such as mental slowing, reduced motivation and low mood – and there appears to be an 'extrapyramidal' component in many persons with dementia: estimates of prevalence of such 'extrapyramidalism' range from 15 per cent to 79 per cent (Knesper 1995).

Case study

Mary was a single lady aged forty-eight affected by Huntington's chorea, which caused severe cognitive and physical impairment and required nursing home care. She had suffered from a depressive illness in her early twenties, possibly triggered by the death of her father from Huntington's. She had again showed signs of depression in her late thirties, but also had signs early signs of dementia. For several years she was very distressed, but in the last two years appeared to lose some insight and became calmer – at least, outwardly. Staff were reporting that she now showed marked restlessness and was prone to crying out. One-to-one care helped at times, but on many occasions seemed to be of no use. She had been given diazepam, but whilst causing no obvious adverse effects, it did not seem to help her. She was then prescribed dothiepin (which she had received in the past). About two weeks after the dose had been increased to 100mg at night she began to be less agitated and this aspect of her condition improved. It was considered that she had probably had a recurrence of depression and that long-term antidepressants were warranted to reduce the risk of relapse.

Although personal intervention did not help in this case, it is important, as ever, to consider non-drug interventions. Psychological interventions such as cognitive therapy have been shown to be of value in depression without dementia (see for example Gloaguen *et al.* 1998), and although evidence is lacking for such therapy in persons with dementia, there is much to suggest reassessment of a person's total care environment, especially his or her interactions with carers, would be of benefit to people with dementia.

The class of drugs called 'antidepressants' is, like anti-psychotics, a chemically diverse group brought together because of traditional clinical usage. They share a common action in terms of brain chemistry, but there is also evidence that they can be of benefit in other syndromes – anxiety, or obsessive-compulsive disorder – and that they show different levels of effectiveness in these other syndromes. Indeed, there is some evidence that serotonin disturbance may be associated not only with depression but also aggression, suggesting another role for 'antidepressants' with a marked serotonin activity.

Antidepressants can be divided into two broad groups: those which block the reuptake of certain neurotransmitters associated with depression, called monoamines; and a second group which inhibits the breakdown of monoamines by an enzyme called monoamine oxidase. Hence the two groups are called, 'Monoamine reuptake inhibitors' (MARIs) and 'monoamine oxidase inhibitors' (MAOIs). MARIs can be further subdivided: less specific, usually older drugs, often referred to as 'tricyclics' by virtue of their chemical structure; and more recent class of drugs which have a more specific effect on the re-uptake of serotonin and are referred to as the Specific Serotonin Reuptake Inhibitors – or SSRIs. There is even a type of drug focused on both serotonin and noradrenaline, i.e. a Serotonin Noradrenaline Reuptake Inhibitor (SNRI).

MAOI's – which cause permanent inhibition of both A and B forms of the enzyme which breaks down monoamine neurotransmitters – are little used generally and rarely in persons with dementia. However, a related class of drug: 'Reversible Inhibitors of Monoamine oxidase A' ('RIMA') has been developed, which has a more specific and less long-term effect. This means that adverse reactions to certain foods or medicines are less of a problem.

This classification is useful in that it allows an appreciation of the range and terminologies of antidepressants. To a degree, understanding side effect profiles and to some extent efficacy profiles – at least, in depressive problems not associated with dementia – can be useful. It should be noted that this approach, strongly influenced by theories of the mode of drug action, is not perfect – not least because all these drugs (even the 'selective' ones) affect other neurotransmitter systems which form a complex, interacting network whose nature is only dimly understood.

EFFICACY

The distinction alluded to above between depressive symptoms, such as unhappiness or agitation, and depressive disorder does appear to impact upon the value of drug treatments. Although in practice diagnosis may not be clear cut, evidence from the treatment of depression in people without dementia would lead to suggestions that the fuller the picture is of a major depressive disorder, the higher the chance of a response to medication. In respect of depressive disorder in persons with dementia, a comprehensive review of evidence about dementia care suggests that the response rate to antidepressants could be as high as 85 per cent (Eccles *et al.* 1998), although the corresponding placebo response rate is not reported and this figure seems optimistic when compared to response rates for people without dementia.

Turning to the wider use of antidepressants in persons with dementia for depressive symptoms, there appear to be few double blind placebo controlled studies and only three further studies concerning more general problems such as agitation or cognitive performance (Lantz and Marin 1996; Roth, Mountjoy and Amrein 1996).

The four placebo controlled studies where patients with depressive symptoms were treated did not yield similar results: a trial of imipramine and maprotiline found that both the placebo treated and antidepressant treated patients improved, with no overall advantage for antidepressants (although maprotiline had a net advantage according to some measures) (Lantz and Marin 1996). In contrast, a study of the selective reuptake inhibitor citalopram did find benefit, as did a study with moclobemide (Roth *et al.* 1996).

Two studies of treatment (with the SSRI's fluvoxamine and alaproclate) for persons with dementia with a wider range of problems such as agitation or irritability showed no benefit (Lantz and Marin 1996).

Although there are some doubts regarding trials without placebo treatment groups, a recent comparative trial of trazodone and haloperidol in the treatment of agitation found both drugs led to an equal overall improvement, but that trazodone was associated with fewer adverse effects, although sedation and low blood pressure (postural hypertension) were reported (Sultzer *et al.* 1997). Of further interest is that improvements with trazodone were noted after seven weeks of treatment, suggesting that simple sedation could not be the factor in such improvements, as sedation would usually be present in the first few days of treatment. This study raises the possibility of less adverse alternatives to antipsychotics in the treatment of agitation.

This is clearly not the occasion to discuss the value of antidepressants in general, but it is worth noting that the efficacy of antidepressants in 'ordinary' depressive episodes is about 60–70 per cent. This compares to a placebo response rate ranging between 30–40 per cent (Silverstone and Turner 1988):

in other words, a net treatment effect of the order of 30 – 40 per cent.

SIDE EFFECTS AND DOSAGES

With so few trials of antidepressants in persons with dementia, there is little direct data on their side effects, so much of what follows is based upon observations in older persons without dementia in the hope that this will apply to dementia suffers, younger as well as older.

The dosage of antidepressants for persons with dementia could be lower for older adults because, although similar blood levels may be required as in younger adults, older persons tend to have higher drug blood levels for a given dose (Alexopoulous 1996: see also pages 30–31 for further discussion). At the same time, under-treatment of depression (especially with low doses of tricyclics) is a common problem, and exposes patients to treatment risks with little chance of treatment benefit: thus, for most tricyclics, eventual doses of less than 100mg daily will not help most recipients. However, because some side effects are more likely when certain antidepressants (most tricyclics) are started, it is usual to commence such antidepressants on a lower dose than the one normally required for response. Anti-depressants can be given in divided doses, or perhaps more easily as one dose (at night, unless insomnia is a potential side effect). General experience with antidepressants would suggest that since a full response to treatment can be delayed by several weeks, treatment should be tried for at least four weeks and preferably eight.

There is no literature on how long antidepressants should be maintained in dementia, nor at what dose. In persons with depressive disorder, research indicates the dose at which response took place should be continued for several months (preferably at least four) before gradual reduction. There is no evidence for addiction to antidepressants, but withdrawal syndromes, caused by sudden cessation, have been described in persons without dementia – again, there is no current research data regarding antidepressant withdrawal problems in dementia. One study suggests that risk of hip fracture is nearly doubled in people taking tricyclic antidepressants, although this study was conducted before the widespread use of the newer antidepressants such as SSRI's, so no data is available for such drugs in this respect (Ray *et al.* 1987). Appendices IV and V list some common antidepressants and interactions respectively.

SUMMARY: ARE ANTIDEPRESSANTS SAFE AND EFFECTIVE?

The fact that depressive problems are so common in dementia underlines the need to consider the use of antidepressant medication, but unfortunately the research evidence suggests that the response rate may be less in comparison to treating typical depressive syndromes. This may well be linked to the physical pathologies of dementia. There is some evidence that antidepressants may be of equal value to antipsychotics in treating agitation. On the whole, these medications are less prone to cause severe side effects than antipsychotics, but problems such as falls and constipation are present, perhaps especially with tricyclic antidepressants. Further research is required and may confirm the impression that newer drugs, such as SSRIs, may cause fewer troublesome side effects.

ANTI-ANXIETY DRUGS

Anxiety is an unavoidable and to some extent essential part of normal life: judging when it is present to abnormal (i.e. excessive) levels is never straightforward, as it remains in essence an inner experience. This can make assessment in persons with dementia somewhat difficult.

Over the years, various substances have been used to reduce anxiety, including alcohol, morphine derivatives and barbiturates. More modern drugs – such as the benzodiazepines (e.g. chlordiazepoxide or oxazepam) became available in the 1960s and it was in that era that the first studies of anti-anxiety agents in dementia were undertaken.

There are several types of anxiolytic agent, which appear to have actions via three different neurotransmitters.

Group one: Benzodiazepines and chloral derivatives

The first type, often referred to as 'minor tranquillizers' is made up of benzodiazepines and chloral derivatives (such as chloral hydrate). These affect brain receptors associated with the neurotransmitter gamma-amino-butyric acid – more easily rendered as GABA. This neurotransmitter depresses (or inhibits) neuronal activity and has a role in arousal, anxiety and proneness to epileptic fits ('seizure threshold') – such that agents promoting GABA action reduce alertness and anxiety, and raise the seizure threshold. Anxiolytics in this class seem to accentuate the effects of GABA (rather than imitate it). Interestingly, substances such as alcohol and barbiturates have comparable effects.

There is much clinical evidence to suggest that all of these substances have an addictive potential – and that withdrawal symptoms from one may be reduced by taking another (e.g. alcohol withdrawal symptoms can be reduced by a benzo-diazepine). There is a related phenomenon of 'tolerance' – that is, after a period of time (perhaps a month or so) drug effects tend to diminish, so a higher dose is required to achieve the same effect. Abrupt withdrawal from any of the drugs in this group is linked to an increased risk of fits. Finally, taking these substances in combination (e.g. alcohol plus benzodiazepines) greatly increases the risk of adverse events such as drowsiness or reduced respiration.

Although there are many available benzodiazepines, the key differences between them lie in the speed of entry into the brain (which may be linked to addictive potential) and the half-life – which is again possibly linked to the risk of addiction, since the shorter the half-life, the more abrupt the withdrawal effects upon stopping the drug. The half-life of drugs is also linked to the risk of accumulation, where a long half-life increases the risk of increasingly high levels of the drug. Appendix VI provides information about some commonly prescribed benzodiazepines.

Group two: Buspirone

The second type of anxiolytic acts upon a different neuro-transmitter system, namely that of serotonin (or 5–HT); there is evidence that serotonin is involved with the functions of GABA described above (Silverstone and Turner 1988). There is one member of this group – buspirone. It has little sedating effect and its action is delayed by the order of several weeks – a similar delay to antidepressants. Indeed, antidepressants do have some efficacy in various anxiety disorders. Quite possibly because of its delayed effect, buspirone does not appear to be addictive. It does not reduce benzodiazepine withdrawal symptoms.

Group three: Beta-blockers

The final group of anxiolytics are called beta-blockers, since they block beta-receptors for the neurotransmitter adrenaline, which is released to excessive levels in anxiety, especially during panic attacks: propanolol is the most often used drug of this type. Beta-blocking agents do not act predominantly in the brain, but rather in parts of the autonomic nervous system (which subconsciously regulates bodily functions). They reduce the physical components of anxiety – such as palpitations or tremor. They are not thought to have much direct psychoactive effect (although there is speculation about some 'central' i.e. brain action) and although their effect is rapid, beta-blockers are not addictive.

The links between dementia and anxiety syndromes or symptoms have not been researched as much as depressive or psychotic symptoms, and the literature concerning the use of these drugs in dementia tends to refer to them as alternative agents to antipsychotics in the reduction of agitation, including aggression.

Benzodiazepines: Efficacy

One of the earliest double blind placebo controlled trials which included persons with dementia was reported in 1965 (Chesrow *et al.*). The trialists compared three treatments: oxazepam, chlordiazepoxide and placebo. The rates of improvement were 56 per cent, 23 per cent and 0 per cent respectively. This study (like so many of its era) included patients with a wide range of problems, probably mainly what might now be called vascular dementia. Whilst subsequent studies may not have reported such clear cut results, several reviewers concur that there is evidence for the efficacy of benzodiazepines in respect of agitation in persons with dementia syndromes (Lantz and Marin 1996; Tariot *et al.* 1995). However, in the light of the associated risks (see below) they are both cautious, and Borson and Rishkind (1997) p.882 conclude 'there is little evidence to support their use as first-line agents'.

Benzodiazepines: Side effects

Whilst these agents do not have the wide range of side effects seen with drugs such as antipsychotics, research suggests that sedation, unsteadiness (with increased risk of falls and fractures), impaired cognitive abilities and occasionally a paradoxical increased agitation are all genuine problems, along with the tolerance and withdrawal phenomena described above. This undoubtedly accounts for reviewers' lack of enthusiasm for these drugs; they suggest that, if used at all, they should only be employed for a short time, up to 8 weeks: this may be because tolerance and withdrawal phenomena tend to develop after such a period.

There does not appear to be much research literature concerning chloral derivatives, there is evidence for a proneness to develop high levels of the drugs, with consequent over-sedation. Barbiturates, with their known marked risks of slowing respiration, dependency and interactions with other drugs, offer no therapeutic advantage over benzodiazepines and would appear to be inappropriate for this group of patients (unless they are being prescribed for epilepsy).

A study has demonstrated about an 80 per cent increased risk of hip fracture with taking long-acting anti-anxiety drugs or sedatives as noted with antipsychotics and antidepressants (Ray *et al.* 1987).

Buspirone

There do not appear to have been any placebo controlled trials of buspirone in dementia-related problems. Some open studies were carried out, and there was one small trial comparing it with the antidepressant trazodone; only the latter gave any improvement (Lantz and Marin 1996). Another reviewer, on the basis of the open studies and case reports, states that buspirone 'appears (to be) effective', but goes on to stress, as do others, the urgent need for controlled trials of this and other newer medications, which are being prescribed with increasing frequency (Borson and Rishkind 1997). The side effects of buspirone are few, but include headache, increased anxiety and dizziness.

Beta-blockers

As with buspirone there has been little research with these agents in persons with dementia-related problems. There are some case series reports of propanolol, and one very small controlled study (of ten patients with a variety of dementia syndromes using a 'cross-over' design): it reported a reduction in aggressiveness (Greendyke *et al.* 1986). This study, with such small numbers and a less than ideal design may not be a reliable indicator of efficacy. Pindolol, a beta-blocker with less side effects than propanolol has been studied under controlled conditions (Lantz and Marin 1996). Two small trials reported a reduction in aggression, but only in one did this difference reach statistical significance.

Side effects include postural hypotension (with dizziness) and worsening of heart failure and of asthma. Confusion and psychotic symptoms have also been reported.

Anxiolytics: Conclusions

There is evidence for treatment efficacy with benzodiazepines, but at with a definite risk of side effects or complications such as sedation, unsteadiness and dependency. Such concerns probably account for reviews which advise caution in prescribing benzodiazepines to persons with dementia for more than eight weeks, or indeed any prescription of them at all. It is interesting to note that the same reviewers tend to reiterate the value of antipsychotic medication, despite noting the somewhat modest efficacy, and concerns regarding potentially severe short- and long-term effects. It is not entirely clear to me why this should be the balance of opinion; perhaps the risks of tolerance and withdrawal phenomena weigh heavily against benzodiazepines.

If a benzodiazepine is tried, perhaps oxazepam, or another short half-life agent such as lorazepam should be considered. These medications are probably best used in divided doses and, as with antipsychotics, timings can be adjusted to vary with any regular patterns of disturbance (e.g. in late afternoon). I am unaware, however, of any research evidence to support this approach (which, for want of repetition, suggests avoidance of any emphatic opinions in a field where placebo effects and variable study outcomes are prominent).

As for buspirone and beta-blockers, it seems to be a case of 'watch this space': these compounds show some promise, but lack of good evidence for efficacy rules them out as front-line treatments, and perhaps beta-blockers (for which the evidence base is rather thin) should only be tried under close supervision and monitoring – for example in nursing homes or hospital care, because of the potential medical problems.

TREATMENTS FOR SLEEPING PROBLEMS

About one-quarter of persons with dementia might have difficulties with sleep (see page 19). This may range from interrupted sleep to a complete reversal of the normal pattern of day and night. However, before prescribing medication for sleep problems a number of steps should be taken. First of all, a check should be made that unrealistic expectations are not being held; for example, if a person is being put to bed at nine in the evening and never slept more than six hours when younger, one could predict difficulties at around three in the morning. Furthermore, older people (in general) sleep less at night (sometimes taking naps during the day); many residential homes will take this into account.

Once a real problem is confirmed, it is important to check for any factors which may account for sleep disturbance, such as pain, urinary frequency or disturbance by others. Other possible considerations include the need to avoid late evening stimulants such as tea or coffee; attempts should be made to establish a regular bed-time and a familiar pattern of activities before going to bed. It is also important to establish that the person themselves is adversely affected by such a change in sleeping pattern, since at least in residential settings it may be possible to work round the problem: for example, it may be better to get up with the person and to keep them occupied, and then take them to bed after half an hour or so, rather than trying to keep them in bed throughout the night. This is not always the case, of course, and for lone carers in their own homes disturbed sleep can be extremely stressful.

If such interventions fail, clinicians may begin to consider the use of sedative drugs, that is hypnotics. There is little specific literature on the drug treatment of sleep problems in persons with dementia, although there is some evidence for the efficacy of benzodiazepines in this context (Tariot *et al.* 1995). Benzodiazepines and chloral derivatives are widely prescribed for sleep disorders. In recent years a new class of sedatives, cyclopyrrolones, has been introduced, which includes drugs such as zopiclone. These appear to act upon the GABA receptor, as do benzodiazepines, but on a different site. They have a short duration of action and are said to be less disruptive of normal sleep patterns than conventional sedatives. I am unaware of any efficacy or side effect data for persons with dementia, but in other persons there is occasional nausea, dizziness, headache and day-time drowsiness.

The same cautions regarding the use of benzodiazepines in agitation apply here: short half-life medications (such as lorazepam) should be tried before longer half-life drugs and should not be prescribed for more than a few weeks at a time. Prescribers might also consider other classes of sedatives such as zopiclone, mentioned above; their addictive potential remains unknown. Sometimes low doses of sedative antidepressants are prescribed for insomnia – but I am unaware of any trial data for the use of such drugs for sleep disorders in this patient group. The various problems attending antipsychotic medication would suggest avoidance of such agents if insomnia is the only major problem – that is, if there is no other disturbance which might merit an antipsychotic. Antihistamines, which tend to be sedative, are sometimes prescribed for insomnia (see also page 104).

MOOD STABILIZERS

Drugs used to reduce the severity and frequency of mood swings in persons with bipolar mood disorder, (including overactivity or aggressiveness in mania) have been studied in persons with agitation or aggression related to dementia. There are two distinct drug groups, one being drugs such as carbamazepine which are also used as anticonvulsants (drugs to treat epilepsy); the second being lithium salts.

Anticonvulsant mood stabilizers

Examples of anticonvulsant mood stabilizers include carbamazepine (Tegretol), which has effects upon serotonin activity and sodium valproate (Epilim), which has a GABA enhancing effect (although not at the same site as benzodiazepines or barbiturates, both of which have useful anticonvulsant, but not mood stabilizing effects).

Efficacy data is not extensive: one double blind placebo controlled trial of carbamazepine showed benefit regarding agitation (using an average 300mg/day dose) – but another (using a *maximal* daily dose of 300mg) showed no benefit (Borson and Rishkind 1997; Lantz and Marin 1996). As is usually the case with drug treatments, case reports and open trials are more optimistic in terms of benefit than controlled trials. In the UK, carbamazepine has an officially listed role as a mood stabilizer for persons with mood disorders, but not for agitation/aggressive problems, or for persons with dementia.

I have no knowledge of any placebo controlled trials of sodium valproate – which in the UK does not have a psychiatric disorder as an official indication for use; case reports indicate a possible benefit.

Side effect information for persons with dementia is similarly scarce: the two treatment trials of carbamazepine reported minimal side effects, but reported side effects in general use include dizziness, headache, unsteady walking, drowsiness, tiredness and nausea (with reports of reduced appetite and weight loss). Because of risks of toxicity, and (rarely) low white blood cell counts, blood levels, liver functions, and full blood counts should be monitored. Carbamazepine can increase ('induce') metabolic liver enzymes and so lower the blood levels of a wide range of drugs, including some other anticonvulsants, some antidepressants and antipsychotics, digoxin and warfarin.

Sodium valproate can produce sedation, unsteadiness and tremor: increased appetite and weight gain are also reported. It has a different, and generally reduced side effect profile as compared to carbamazepine, but monitoring of blood levels, liver function and pre-treatment full blood counts are still advised. Again as with carbamazepine, metabolic enzyme induction can reduce the effect of other drugs, but this problem is less marked with sodium valproate.

Lithium salts

Lithium salts, of which one example is lithium carbonate (Priadel), are widely used in persons with mood disorders, especially those with a history of manic episodes. There have been studies of their use for aggression in other patient groups, but there appear to be only case reports and one case series of ten concerning persons with dementia (Borson and Rishkind 1997). These reports are somewhat mixed, with the case series finding no benefit. Lithium has relatively few side effects, but there are significant risks of toxicity and effects upon the heart, kidneys and thyroid glands which require pre-treatment tests and continued monitoring (requirements which, apart from the lack clear efficacy, suggest that lithium would be an unusual treatment for persons with dementia).

MOOD STABILIZERS: CONCLUSIONS

There may be a role for anticonvulsants such as carbamazepine or sodium valproate, but these drugs do have some complications in terms of drug interactions and possible toxicity, so further evidence of efficacy would be desirable before their widespread adoption into routine practice. There is scant evidence for any benefit from lithium salts and their toxicity problems and the associated monitoring requirements would appear to make them unsuitable for clinical use and potentially problematic for inclusion in treatment trials.

OTHER TREATMENTS
Antihistamines

Antihistamines such as diphenhydramine have been prescribed to relieve agitation in dementia. The rationale behind this is largely based on the sedative properties of antihistamines. (The antipsychotic chlorpromazine was discovered as one of a series of compounds being tested as candidate antihistamines and the sedative properties of antipsychotics are strongly linked to their blocking action of histamine.) Coccaro *et al.* (1990) conducted a comparative trial of diphenhydramine with haloperidol and oxazepam. They describe improvement in all three treatment groups, but no statistically significant differences were found, although the impact of both haloperidol and diphenhydramine appeared to exceed that of oxazepam. This study lacked a placebo group, which, as mentioned before, renders application to general clinical practice difficult. Antihistamines are prone to cause excessive sedation, anticholinergic side effects (such as dry mouth, blurred vision and constipation) and have a number of interactions with other drugs.

Oestrogens

There are case reports of the use of oestrogens in reducing aggression with a sexual component in males with dementia. I am unaware of any controlled studies and there may well be ethical issues around the use of such compounds in persons who cannot adequately consent to treatment (Lantz and Marin 1996).

Chapter 8

Drugs Treatments and Dementia

Summing Up

EMERGING THEMES

Looking at the evidence about drug treatments in dementia over-all, it does seem that with the exception of treatment of depression, drug efficacy is generally at a modest level, whether in respect of antipsychotics and agitation, antidepressants and depressive symptoms or cholinesterase inhibitors and cognitive performance (the benefits of the latter being even more mar-ginal). Furthermore, the recurring problem in appraising the evidence for drug treatments for people with dementia is how to gauge their overall impact: this makes it hard for readers of such studies to find out really useful information when making treat-ment decisions. Allied to this, the focus of most research upon the individual as a patient, rather than as a person living within their own social context, runs the risk of engendering a narrow approach to care interventions which could miss vital steps in understanding and helping.

This is not perhaps welcome news to pressured care staff or primary care clinicians who might desire a rapid 'solution' to what can feel like overwhelming difficulties – especially when a particular person is by no means the only client presenting challenging or even dangerous problems. In a different vein, there can be few people involved with people who have dementia who do not hope for a definitive cure, or at least a treatment which will halt decline at a very early stage. So new treatments enter upon a scene of great hope and high emotion.

The reasons why dementia drug treatments are of such modest benefit are not clear, but could include the brute fact of neuronal damage and death; also that dementia affects a wide range of neurotransmitters, so drugs whose beneficial effects are linked to a particular neurotransmitter would seem to have limited scope for success. Perhaps another reason is that non-biological factors – such as interactions with carers – have a very important part to play, so reducing the relative advantage of 'active' treatments over placebo.

There also seems to be evidence that treatments do not necessarily follow their classical role in terms of efficacy – thus 'antidepressants' may be as effective as haloperidol in reducing agitation, and 'cognitive enhancers' may have antipsychotic properties. The 'psychobehavioural metaphor' approach (see page 23) may retain some value, but perhaps these analogies will appear less useful as more is learnt about the actions and efficacies of drug treatments and the interplay between neurotransmitter systems and psychosocial factors.

Another common theme, though not a universal one, is the presence of troublesome and sometimes dangerous side effects. These two themes – small treatment effects and risks of adverse events – should surely lead to careful consideration before embarking upon drug treatments, and vigilance in monitoring their effects.

Caution seems to be most warranted in respect of conventional antipsychotics: as stated already, drugs which appear only to help 20 per cent of their recipients, yet cause significant side effects – some potentially persistent – in 50 per cent of patients should clearly be used as a matter of last resort. (Readers may also be aware of a wider debate around the side effects and use of conventional antipsychotics in other conditions, such as schizophrenia.) As for novel antipsychotics, these may be of value in dementia-related problems – but further research is required before their inclusion into routine practice.

I would echo the restraint advised by recent reviewers in rushing to embrace other psychotropic medications whose efficacy and safety in dementia-related problems is yet to be established. Thus, the 1987 study by Ray *et al.* concerning the risks of hip fracture is often cited to show the hazards of antipsychotics (about a two-fold increased risk of fracture). Yet the risk associated with tricyclic antidepressants and longer-acting sedatives were almost as high. This lends some weight to the very cautious use of antipsychotics in very specific situations – such as where psychotic symptoms are evident or, perhaps, when there are serious risks and other measures have failed.

Turning to the new dementia treatments, there can be no denying the excitement such advances can bring, with the prospects for really effective anti-dementia treatment not seeming nearly so remote. Clearly this is a fast changing scene, but although the new cognitive enhancers such as donepezil and rivastigmine do represent some advance, they nonetheless are symptomatic treatments with only modest benefits for a minority of patients. Given the (justifiable) requirements for drugs to have demonstrable efficacy and safety before receiving approval, it looks as though major therapeutic advances are still some way down the road. The possibility that demonstrable cost-effectiveness will be an additional requirement for approval should help to rationalize decisions about health care priorities, so long as dementia treatments are not singled out for such an approach and that there is not undue delay in clinically valuable treatments becoming available.

SOME GUIDELINES FOR DRUG TREATMENT

Putting all of the evidence together, how should a clinician – say a primary care physician – respond when asked to prescribe for a person with dementia? The summary sections in the foregoing chapters will provide more detailed advice, but some overall guidance is given below, with the usual 'health warning' regarding the limits of such guidance, since at the end of the day all treatment decisions are made by individual clinicians working with colleagues and (hopefully) considering options with the person themselves and their carers.

First, if there was to be one message to emerge from this guide, it would be that *drug treatment for persons with dementia should never be commenced without a careful appraisal of a person's whole situation and the likely balance between overall benefit and adversity for that individual.* Indeed, most clinicians who work with people who have dementia would concur that *drugs have at most a small role within overall care.* By and large, it is excessive drug treatment, rather than under treatment, which is the problem for persons with dementia.

Second, if depression appears to be present, then alongside other interventions, a full treatment trial of antidepressant medication should be considered. This means treatment with at least the minimum effective dose for at least four weeks. The responsiveness of isolated depressive symptoms, such as fleeting low mood, is less clear cut.

Third, the problem of agitation (including restlessness and aggression) can be very taxing for carers and often seems to lead to pressure to 'do something' (by contrast, withdrawal or lethargy may attract much less concern). This review of evidence (and others, e.g. Eccles *et al.* 1998) points away from antipsychotic medication as the drug treatment of first choice (indeed the literature points away from the use of medication wherever possible, unless perhaps there are distressing psychotic symptoms, in which case a trial course of a few weeks might be in order). But if drugs are to be used for agitation or aggression, what alternatives are there? Perhaps trials should be made with anti-depressants or anxiolytics – although only the problematic benzodiazepines have much evidence to support their use.

Fourth, the value of new treatments such as donepezil or rivastigmine is not fully established, but – depending on local arrangements – trials of treatment with all parties being well informed about the fairly low chance of a positive response may be justifiable in persons with mild or moderate dementia in Alzheimer's disease. Probably such trials should only be conducted by specialists with expertise in dementia care, such as psychiatrists for older adults or geriatricians. Regarding treatments for underlying dementia pathologies, only aspirin for persons with vascular dementia appears to be of established value.

RESEARCH – FINAL COMMENTS AND FUTURE HOPES

This book has tried to incorporate research findings into guiding treatment decisions, so I will end it with a personal observation that there is something of a paradox about research into drug treatments for persons with dementia. On the one hand, the field of cognitive enhancers and other antidementia agents is one of the largest and fastest moving areas of medical science, with significant developments on almost a monthly basis. I certainly wish such endeavours well, yet in other areas – including those concerning the most common treatments, little research has ever been undertaken and the pace of advance often seems to be measured in decades. The massive imbalance between funding for drug- centred research on the one hand, and research into psycho- social approaches is a further issue. Perhaps the growing interest in dementia which the new treatments have generated will also highlight other concerns about dementia care and drug treatments and so reverse the long years of relative neglect.

Overview of Antipsychotic Side Effects

Blockade of	Resulting side-effect:
Dopamine	extra-pyramidal effects reports of dysphoria (unpleasant or low mood); agitation and anxiety
Acetylcholine	impaired cognitive function / confusion, dry mouth, blurred vision, constipation, retention of urine, fast heart rate
Histamine	sedation; also impaired cognitive function weight gain (but some evidence of weight loss in elderly)
alpha-2 adrenaline	falling blood pressure on standing (postural hypotension), hypothermia
Other effects	
effects on the heart	impaired electrical conduction within the heart, with risk of abnormal heart beat.
rare adverse events	neuroleptic malignant syndrome (muscle rigidity, severe fluctuations of blood pressure and body temperature, with risk of death) skin sensitivity and pigmentation (more common with high dose phenothiazines) low white cell count (leading to decreased resistance to infections)

Names, Side Effects and Dosages of some Antipsychotic Drugs

Name	Side Effects			Suggested Starting Dose
(example UK trade name)	Extra-pyramidal	Anti cholinergic	Sedation	(total daily)
chlorpromazine (Largactil) (1)	+ +	+ +	+ + +	30mg
thioridazine (Melleril) (2)	+	+ + +	+ + +	30mg
trifluoperazine (Stelazine)	+ + +	+	+ +	1mg
haloperidol (Haldol)	+ + +	+	+	1mg
sulpiride (Dolmatil) (3)	+	0	+	200mg
Sources: Tyrer, Harrison-Read and Van Horn 1997; Wood and Castleton 1991; The Association of the British Pharmaceutical Industry 1998.				

Also *olanzapine* (4) and *risperidone* (5): little data available for this client group

(1)   *Chlorpromazine:* higher risk of liver and blood abnormalities and skin sensitivities. *Promazine* (Sparine) is a similar drug.

(2)   *Thioridazine:* widely prescribed for dementia related problems as it is fairly sedating but without marked parkinsonian effects. However, this is at the cost of anticholinergic effects and proneness to cause anti-adrenergic side effects such as low blood pressure.

(3)   *Sulpiride:* a new but not entirely 'novel' antipsychotic, as it has some extra-pyramidal effects. There is some suggestion of a lower risk of tardive dyskinesia.

(4)   *Olanzapine:* a novel antipsychotic with minimal extra-pyramidal side effects (but does cause other side effects such as sedation and dizziness). Of potential value – but there is minimal data regarding use in dementia.

(5)   *Risperidone:* Another new antipsychotic, but it is debatable as to whether it is 'novel', because although it has a therapeutic serotonin blocking action, it also has dopamine blocking effects. At low doses (below 6–8 mg daily) it is effective against schizophrenia but without marked parkinsonian effects: at higher doses, however, these become as frequent as with 'conventional' drugs. There is no control trial data available for treatment in dementia.

Appendix III

Interactions with Antipsychotics

Drug group	Interaction with Antipsychotics
antidepressants	metabolism may be inhibited, raising antidepressant levels
alcohol, barbiturates, other sedatives	increased risk of over sedation and slowed respiration
anticholinergic drugs (e.g. procyclidine)	reduced absorption due to slowed emptying of stomach; possible reduction of antipsychotic effect
antiparkinsonian agents	reduction of anti-parkinsonian effect
anticonvulsants	increased enzyme activity (by anticonvulsants) may lower antipsychotic level
antihypertensives	exaggeration of hypotensive (low blood pressure) effects
antacids	reduced absorption of antipsychotic

Appendix IV

Side Effects and Dosages of Antidepressants

Class	Name	Side Effects			Dosage (mg)
		anti-cholinergic *	sedation	other	starting dose (target dose)
MARI					
tricyclics	amitriptyline (Tryptizol, Lentizol)	+++	+++	heart problems (toxic in overdose) low blood pressure, increased confusion	25 (50–100)
	imipramine (Tofranil)	+++	+++	as for amitriptyline	10 (30–50)
tricyclic-new	lofepramine (Gamanil)	+	rare	side effects less than older tricyclics but still reported; much less toxic in overdose	140 (140–210)
SSRIs	fluoxetine (Prozac)	rare	occ.	nausea, sweating, agitation, insomnia, weight loss: low toxicity	20*** (20)
	citalopram (Cipramil)	rare	occ.	as for fluoxetine	20 (20)
	sertraline (Lustral)	rare	occ.	as for fluoxetine	50 (50)
SNRI	venlafaxine (Efexor)	rare	rare	nausea, headache, insomnia	75 (75–140)
Other	trazodone (Molipaxin)	+	+++	postural hypotension	50–100 (100–300)

Sources: Wood et al. 1991; Silverstone and Turner 1988; The Association of the British Pharmaceutical Industry 1998.

*   anticholinergic side effects include dry mouth, blurred vision, constipation and urinary retention.

**   heart problems: disorders of electrical activity in the heart, with risk of abnormal heart beat; also risk of worsening heart failure.

***   initial dose of fluoxetine: some clinicians advise that with alerting SSRIs such as fluoxetine a lower starting dosage (e.g. 10mg) may reduce the risk of the listed side effects – which, when severe, are recognized as a 'serotonin syndrome'.

Appendix V

Interactions with Antidepressants

All antidepressants	
antipsychotics	inhibition of metabolism leads to increased antidepressant levels
MARI+MAOIs	increased risks of adverse events if any MARI is prescribed with an MAOI
Tricyclics:	
sedatives, barbiturates	increased risk of oversedation: possible reduced effect with barbiturates
SSRIs	
lithium	alteration of lithium levels; reports of toxicity

Characteristics of some Benzodiazepines

benzodiazepine	speed of action	half-life	initial daily dosage
diazepam (Valium)	rapid	long: 20–45 hrs*	2mg
nitrazepam (Mogadon)	medium	long	5mg
temazepam (Normison)	rapid	short	10mg
lorazepam (Ativan)	rapid	short	0.5–1mg
oxazepam (Serenid)	medium	short	30mg

Sources: Silverstone and Turner 1988; Tyrer et al. 1997; The Association of British Pharmaceutical Industry 1998.

* the effective half-life of diazepam is 50–100 hours, when active metabolites are included; neither lorazepam nor oxazepam have active metabolites.

References

Alexopoulos, G.S. (1996) 'The treatment of depressed demented patients.' *Journal of Clinical Psychiatry, 57,* Suppl 14,14–20.

Association of the British Pharmaceutical Industry (1998) *ABPI Compendium of Data Sheets and Summaries of Product Characteristics.* London: Datapharm Publications Ltd.

Barton, R. and Hurst, L. (1966) 'Unnecessary use of tranquillisers in elderly patients.' *British Journal of Psychiatry, 112,* 989–990.

Birks, J. and Melzer, D. (1998) 'The efficacy of donepezil for mild and moderate Alzheimer's disease.' *Cochrane Database of Systematic Reviews.* In Cochrane Library CD ROM.

Borson, S. and Doane, K. (1997) 'The Impact of OBRA-87 on Psychotropic Drug Prescribing in Skilled Nursing Facilities.' *Psychiatric Services, 48,* 10, 1289–1296.

Borson, S. and Rishkind, M.A. (1997) 'Clinical features and pharmacologic treatment of behavioral symptoms of Alzheimer's disease.' *Neurology, 48,* Suppl 6, S17–S24.

Breitner, J.C., Gau, B.A., Welsh, K.A., Plassman, B.L., McDonald, W.M., Helms, M.J. and Anthony, J.C. (1994) 'Inverse association of anti-inflammatory treatments and Alzheimer's disease: Initial results of a co-twin study.' *Neurology, 44,* 20, 227–232.

Bridges-Parlet, S., Knopman, D. and Steffes, S. (1997) 'Withdrawal of neuroleptic medications from institutionalized dementia patients: Results of a double-blind, baseline-treatment-controlled pilot study.' *Journal of Geriatric Psychiatry and Neurology, 10,* 119–126.

Burke, W.J. (1991) 'Neuroleptic drug use in the nursing home: The impact of OBRA-87.' *American Family Physician, 43,* 6, 2125–2130.

Chesrow, E.J., Kaplitz, S.E., Vetra, H., Breme, J.T. and Marquardt, G.H. (1965) 'Blind study of oxazepam in the management of geriatric patients with behavioural problems.' *Clinical Medicine,* 1001–1005.

Coccaro, E.F., Kramer, E., Zemishlany, Z., Thorne, A., Rice, M., Giordani, B., Duvvi, K., Patel, B.M., Torres, J., Nora, R., Neufeld, R., Mohs, R.C. and Davis, K.L. (1990) 'Pharmacologic treatment of noncognitive behavioural disturbances in elderly demented patients.' *American Journal of Psychiatry, 147,* 12, 1640–1645.

Cohen-Mansfield, J. (1986) 'Agitated behaviors in the elderly II: Preliminary results in the cognitively deteriorated.' *Journal of the American Geriatric Society, 34,* 722–727.

Cohen-Mansfield, J. and Billig, N. (1986) 'Agitated Behaviors in the Elderly I: A Conceptual Review.' *Journal of the American Geriatrics Society, 34,* 711–721.

Consumers' Association (1998) 'Donepezil Update.' *Drug and Therapeutic Bulletin, 36,* 8, 60–61.

Corey-Bloom, J., Anand, R. and Veach, J. for the ENA 713 B352 Study Group (1998) 'A randomised trial evaluating the efficacy and safety of ENA 713 (rivastigmine tartrate), a new acetylcholinesterase inhibitor, in patients with mild to moderately severe Alzheimer's disease.' *International Journal of Geriatric Psychopharmacology, 1,* 55–65.

Covert, A.B., Rodrigues, T. and Solomon, K. (1977) 'The use of mechanical and chemical restraints in nursing homes.' *Journal of the American Geriatrics Society, 25,* 2, 85–89.

Cummings, J.L. and Kaufer, D. (1996) 'Neuropsychiatric aspects of Alzheimer's disease: The cholinergic hypothesis revisited.' *Neurology, 47,* 876–883.

de la Torre, J.C. (1997) 'Cerebromicrovascular pathology in Alzheimer's disease compared to normal aging.' *Gerontology, 43,* 1–2, 26–43.

Devanand, D.P. and Levy, S.R. (1995) 'Neuroleptic treatment of agitation and psychosis in dementia.' *Journal of Geriatric Psychiatry and Neurology, 8,* suppl 1, S18–S27.

Devasenapathy, A. and Hachinski, V. (1997) 'Vascular cognitive impairment: A new approach.' In C. Holmes and R. Howard (eds) *Advances in Old Age Psychiatry – Chromosomes to Community Care.* Petersfield and Bristol, PA: Wrightson Biomedical Publishing.

Eccles, M., Clarke, J., Livingstone, M., Freemantle, N. and Mason, J. for the North of England Evidence Based Dementia Guideline Development Group (1998) 'North of England evidence based guidelines development project: Guidelines for the primary care management of dementia.' *British Medical Journal, 317,* 802–808.

Esiri, M. (1991) 'Neuropathology.' In R. Jacoby and C. Oppenheimer (eds) *Psychiatry in the Elderly.* Oxford: Oxford University Press.

Folstein, M.F., Folstein, S.E. and McHugh, P.R. (1975) '"Mini-Mental State": A practical method for grading the cognitive state of subjects for the clinician.' *Journal of Psychiatric Research, 12,* 189–198.

Gloaguen, V., Cottraux, J., Cucherat, M. and Blackburn, I.-M. (1998) 'A meta-analysis of the effects of cognitive therapy in depressed patients.' *Journal of Affective Disorders, 49,* 59–72.

Greendyke, R.M., Kanter, D.R., Schuster, D.B., Verstreate, S. and Wootton, J. (1986) 'Propanolol treatment of assaultative patients with organic brain disease. A bouble-blind crossover, placebo-controlled study.' *Journal of Nervous and Mental Disease, 174,* 5, 290–294.

Guscott, R. and Taylor, L. (1994) 'Lithium prophylaxis in recurrent affective illness: Efficacy, effectiveness and efficiency.' *British Journal of Psychiatry, 164,* 741–746.

Henderson, A.S., Jorm, A.F., Christensen, H., Jacomb, P.A. and Korten, A.E. (1997) 'Aspirin, anti-inflammatory drugs and risk of dementia.' *International Journal of Geriatric Psychiatry, 12,* 926–930.

Hinchliffe, A.C., Katona, C. and Livingston, G. (1997) 'The assessment and management of behavioural manifestations of dementia: a review and results of a controlled trial.' *International Journal of Psychiatry in Clinical Practice, 1,* 157–168.

Hirsch, C.H. (1997) 'Selegiline or alpha-tocopherol slowed the progression of Alzheimer disease.' (commentary) *Evidence-Based Medicine,* November/December (Therapeutics), 175.

Kirchner, V., Kelly, C.A. and Harvey, R.J. (1998) 'A systematic review of the evidence for the safety and efficacy of thioridazine in dementia.' *Cochrane Database of Systematic Reviews.* In Cochrane Library CD ROM.

Kitwood, T. (1997) *Dementia Reconsidered: The Person Comes First.* Buckingham: Open University Press.

Kitwood, T. and Bredin, K. (1992) 'A new approach to the evaluation of dementia care.' *Journal of Advances in Health and Nursing Care, 1,* 5, 41–60.

Kleijnen, J. and Knipschild, P. (1992) 'Ginkgo biloba for cerebral insufficiency.' *British Journal of Clinical Pharmacology, 34,* 4, 252–258.

Knesper, D.J. (1995) 'The depressions of Alzheimer's disease: sorting, pharmacotherapy, and clinical advice.' *Journal of Geriatric Psychiatry and Neurology, 8,* suppl. 1, S40–S51.

Lantz, M.S. and Marin, D. (1996) 'Pharmacologic treatment of agitation in dementia: A comprehensive review.' *Journal of Geriatric Psychiatry and Neurology*, 9, 107–119.

Le Bars, P.L., Katz, M.M., Berman, N., Itil, T.M., Freedman, A.M. and Schatzberg, A.F. for the North American EGb Study Group (1997) 'A placebo-controlled, double-blind, randomized trial of an extract of ginkgo biloba for dementia.' *Journal of the American Medical Association*, 278, 16, 1327–1332.

McGrath, A.M. and Jackson, G. (1997) 'Survey of neuroleptic prescribing in residents of nursing homes in Glasgow.' *British Medical Journal*, 312, 611–612.

McShane, R., Keene, J., Gedling, K., Jacoby, R. and Hope, T. (1997) 'Do neuroleptic drugs hasten cognitive decline in dementia? Prospective study with necropsy follow up.' *British Medical Journal*, 314, 266–70.

Mann, A.H., Graham, N. and Ashby, D. (1986) 'The prescription of psychotropic medication in local authority old people's homes.' *International Journal of Geriatric Psychiatry*, 1, 25–29.

Marcusson, J., Rother, M., Kittner, B., Rössner, M., Smith, R.J., Babic, T., Folnegovic-Smalc, V., Möller, H.J. and Labs, K.H. on behalf of the European Propentophylline Study Group (1997) 'A 12-month, randomized, placebo-controlled trial of propentophylline (HWA 285) in patients with dementia according to DSM III-R.' *Dementia and Geriatric Cognitive Disorders*, 8, 320–328.

Patel, V. and Hope, T. (1993) 'Aggressive behaviour in elderly people with dementia: a review.' *International Journal of Geriatric Psychiatry*, 8, 457–472.

Pollock, B.G. and Mulsant, B.H. (1995) 'Antipsychotics in older patients – a safety perspective.' *Drugs and Aging*, 6, 4, 312–323.

Post, S.G. (1998) 'The fear of forgetfulness: a grassroots approach to an ethics of Alzheimer's disease.' *Journal of Clinical Ethics*, 9, 1, 71–79.

Proctor, A.W. (1997) 'Principles of drug treatment in Alzheimer's disease.' In C. Holmes and R. Howard (eds) *Advances in Old Age Psychiatry – Chromosomes to Community Care*. Petersfield and Bristol, PA: Wrightson Biomedical Publishing.

Qizilbash, N., Birks, J., Arrieta, J.L., Lewington, S. and Szeto, S. (1997) 'Tacrine in Alzheimer's: The efficacy of tacrine in Alzheimer's disease.' *Cochrane database of Systematic Reviews*. In Cochrane Library CD ROM.

Qizilbash, N., Arrieta, J.L. and Birks, J. (1997) 'Nimodipine in the treatment of primary degenerative, mixed and vascular dementia.' *Cochrane Database of Systematic Reviews*. In Cochrane Library CD ROM.

Ray, W.A., Federspiel, C.F. and Schaffner, W. (1980) 'A study of antipsychotic drug use in nursing homes: epidemiologic evidence suggesting misuse.' *American Journal of Public Health*, 70, 5, 485–491.

Ray, W.A., Griffin, M.R., Schaffner, W., Baugh, D.K. and Melton, L.J. (1987) 'Psychotropic drug use and the risk of hip fracture.' *New England Journal of Medicine*, 316, 7, 363–368.

Ray, W.A., Taylor, J.A., Meador, K.G., Lichtenstein, M.J., Griffin, M.R., Fought, R., Adams, M.L. and Blazer, D.G. (1993) 'Reducing antipsychotic drug use in nursing homes: A controlled trial of provider education.' *Archives of Internal Medicine*, 153, 713–721.

Risse, S.C. and Barnes, R. (1986) 'Pharmacologic treatment of agitation associated with dementia.' *Journal of the American Geriatrics Society*, 34, 368–376.

Rogers, S.L., Farlow, M.R., Doody, R.S., Mohs, R., Friedhoff, L.T. and the Donepezil Study Group (1998) 'A 24–week, double-blind, placebo-controlled trial of donepezil in patients with Alzheimer's disease.' *Neurology*, 50, 136–145.

Rogers, S.L., Friedhoff, L.T. and the Donepezil Study Group (1996) 'The efficacy and safety of donepezil in patients with Alzheimer's disease: Results of a US multicentre, randomized, double-blind, placebo-controlled trial.' *Dementia, 7,* 293–303.

Roth, M., Mountjoy, C.Q. and Amrein, R. (1996) 'Moclobemide in elderly patients with cognitive decline and depression: an international double-blind, placebo-controlled trial.' *British Journal of Psychiatry, 168,* 2, 149–157.

Sano, M., Ernesto, C. and Thomas, R.G. for the members of the Alzheimer's Disease Cooperative Study (1997) 'A controlled trial of selegiline, alpha-tocopherol, or both as treatment for Alzheimer's disease.' *New England Journal of Medicine, 336,* 1216–1222.

Schneider, L.S. and Olin, J.Y. (1994) 'Overview of clinical trials of hydergine in dementia.' *Archives of Neurology, 51,* 8, 787–798.

Schneider, L.S., Pollock, V.E. and Lyness, S.A. (1990) 'A meta-analysis of controlled trials of neuroleptic treatment in dementia.' *Journal of the American Geriatrics Society, 38,* 553–563.

Schneider, L.S., Pollock, V.E. and Lyness, S.A. (1991) 'Further analysis of a meta-analysis (letter).' *Journal of the American Geriatrics Society, 39,* 4, 441–442.

Silverstone, T. and Turner, P. (1988) *Drug Treatment in Psychiatry.* London: Routledge.

Stürmer, T., Glynn, R.J., Field, T.S., Taylor, J.O. and Hennekens, C.H. (1996) 'Aspirin use and cognitive function in the elderly.' *American Journal of Epidemiology, 143,* 7, 683–691.

Sultzer, D.L., Gray, K.F., Gunay, I., Berisford, A. and Mahler, M.E. (1997) 'A double-blind comparison of trazodone and haloperidol for treatment of agitation in patients with dementia.' *The American Journal of Geriatric Psychiatry, 5,* 1, 60–69.

Sweet, R.A., Pollock, B.G., Rosen, J., Mulsant, B.H., Altieri, L.P. and Perel, J.M. (1994) 'Early detection of neuroleptic-induced parkinsonism in elderly patients with dementia.' *Journal of Geriatric Psychiatry and Neurology, 7,* 251–253.

Tariot, P.N. (1996) 'Treatment strategies for agitation and psychosis in dementia.' *Journal of Clinical Psychiatry, 57,* suppl. 14, 21–29.

Tariot, P.N., Schneider, L.S. and Katz, I.R. (1995) 'Anticonvulsant and other non-neuroleptic treatment of agitation in dementia.' *Journal of Geriatric Psychiatry and Neurology, 8,* suppl. 1, S28–S39.

Thapa, P.B., Meador, K.G., Gideon, P., Fought, R.L. and Ray, W.A. (1994) 'Effects of antipsychotic withdrawal in elderly nursing home residents.' *Journal of the American Geriatric Society, 42,* 280–286.

Tyrer, P., Harrison-Read, P. and Van Horn, E. (1997) *Drug Treatment in Psychiatry.* Oxford: Butterworth-Heinmann.

Wadworth, A.N. and Crisp, P. (1992) 'Co-dergine mesylate. A review of its pharmacodynamic and pharmacokinetic properties and therapeutic use in age-related cognitive decline.' *Drugs and Aging, 2,* 3, 153–173.

Waxman, H.M., Klein, M. and Carner, E. (1985) 'Drug misuse in nursing homes: an institutional addiction?' *Hospital and Community Psychiatry, 36,* 8, 886–887.

Wills, P., Claesson, C.B., Fratiglioni, L., Fastbom, J., Thorslund, M. and Winblad, B. (1997) 'Drug use by demented and non-demented people.' *Age and Ageing, 26,* 5, 383–391.

Wood, P. and Castleton, C.M. (1991) 'Psychopharmacology in the elderly.' In R. Jacoby and C. Oppenheimer (eds) *Psychiatry in the Elderly.* Oxford: Oxford University Press.

Further Reading

Professor Kitwood's *Dementia Reconsidered* (see reference list above) provides a critique of common assumptions about dementia and an accessible discussion of some important ethical and clinical issues, with the interesting suggestion that new approaches to dementia care might be usefully applied in other fields of mental health practice.

Tyrer *et al.*'s *Drug Treatment in Psychiatry* (cited above) is an up-to-date general guide to this field, providing further details of drug actions and pharmacology, as well as including a chapter concerning treatment of organic disorders.

There are a number of books concerning evidence-based approaches to medicine of which a widely regarded example is *Evidence-Based Medicine* by D.L. Sackett, W.S. Richardson, W. Rosenburg and R.B Haynes (1997). London: Churchill Livingston.

For more information about research methodology – of the quantitative type used in most of the reference studies – readers may find *Research Methods in Psychiatry: A Beginner's Guide* by C. Freeman and P. Tyrer (1992) London: Gaskell, a useful text which covers many other aspects than were touched upon in this text.

Subject Index

Author Index

128   DRUGS TREATMENTS AND DEMENTIA